Study Guide to accompany

MEDICAL-SURGICAL NURSING

A Nursing Process Approach

SECOND EDITION

BARBARA C. LONG, M.S.N., R.N.

WILMA J. PHIPPS, Ph.D., R.N., F.A.A.N.

Prepared by

MARY SAYER NICHOLS, R.N., M.S.

Assistant Professor, Medical-Surgical Nursing
Bethune-Cookman College
Daytona Beach, Florida

The C. V. Mosby Company

ST. LOUIS · BALTIMORE · PHILADELPHIA · TORONTO 1989

Mosby

Editor: Linda L. Duncan
Assistant editor: Susie H. Baxter
Project manager: Suzanne Seeley
Book and cover designer: Gail Morey Hudson

Printed in the United States of America

The C. V. Mosby Company
11830 Westline Industrial Drive, St. Louis, Missouri 63146

International Standard Book Number 0-8016-5494-7

PC/PC/PC 9 8 7 6 5 4 3 2 1

Contributors

BRENDA GOODNER, R.N., M.S.N.
Psychotherapist in Private Practice
Santa Teresa, New Mexico
El Paso, Texas

CAROLE KAUFMAN, M.S., C.N.M., A.R.N.P.
Assistant Professor, Maternal and Child-Health
Bethune-Cookman College
Daytona Beach, Florida

JACQUELINE S. SPRAGUE, R.N., M.Ed.
Instructor, Medical-Surgical Nursing
Bethune-Cookman College
Daytona Beach, Florida

VIVIENNE I. WALTON, R.N., M.S.N.
Assistant Professor, Psychiatric Nursing
Psychiatric Clinical Specialist
Bethune-Cookman College
Daytona Beach, Florida

Preface

Nurses have independent and interdependent functions. Therefore, students in any entry level nursing program must learn how to make independent decisions to provide safe care to patients.

Learning is an independent, lifelong process. Thus nursing students at any entry level need to be provided with structured methods and materials to facilitate the development of an attitude of independent learning throughout the educational process.

A student-oriented study guide for Long-Phipps: *Medical-Surgical Nursing* has been developed to foster independent student learning and to promote student accountability in the educational process. The study guide contains 42 chapters, each written to correlate with a specific chapter in Long-Phipps: *Medical-Surgical Nursing,* second edition. Each chapter contains objectives, prerequisite readings, self-assessment activities, and supplemental activities. An answer key is provided for selected self-assessment activities.

Self-assessment activities include defining selected terms, answering multiple choice, true/false, and sentence completion questions, filling in charts, and labeling diagrams. Supplemental activities include suggested readings, group activities, and community activities. Ideas for research have been included in selected chapters as well as case studies, nursing care plans, and teaching plans.

To use the study guide, students should review the objectives and complete the prerequisite readings, then proceed with the self-assessment activities to evaluate their individual learning. We hope this study guide will help the student improve performance on written examinations and serve as a structured means for self-review of medical-surgical nursing content in preparation for the licensure examination.

Please remember to answer the sections in your text chapters, "Putting knowledge to practice," included by the authors of the text.

Contents

UNIT I Medical-Surgical Nursing Practice

Chapter 1

Perspectives of Medical-Surgical Nursing

MARY S. NICHOLS

CHAPTER OBJECTIVES

On completion of this chapter, the student should be able to:

- Differentiate the practice of medical-surgical nursing from the other disciplines (for example, pediatric, psychiatric).
- Differentiate between health promotion and prevention of illness and describe the three levels of prevention.
- Define "at risk" status and explain the relevance for nursing practice.
- Differentiate between illness and disease and identify stages of disease development.
- Identify actions people take when illness is perceived.
- Describe the "sick role."
- Describe the scope of medical-surgical nursing practice: independent and interdependent functions, use of specific knowledge (pathophysiology, signs and symptoms, medical therapies), and types of nursing interventions.

PREREQUISITE READING

Long-Phipps, Chapter 1, pp. 3-10.

SELF-ASSESSMENT ACTIVITIES

I. Define the following terms.

At-risk status
Disease
Epidemiology
Etiology
Health
Health care
Illness
Independent nursing action
Interdependent nursing action
Medical care
Medical-surgical nursing
Mental health
Multiple causality
Noncompliance
Optimal health
Pathophysiology
Pathopsychologic
Primary prevention
Secondary prevention
Sick role
Signs
Symptoms
Tertiary prevention

Terminology used with disease

Acute
Chronic
Course
Incidence
Intervention
Morbidity
Onset
Prognosis
Resolution
Spontaneous
Therapeutic

II. Briefly discuss the following concepts.

1. Describe the primary focus of medical-surgical nursing.

2. Give some examples of activities directed toward helping persons maintain a high level of well-being.

3. Define prevention.

4. Differentiate among primary, secondary, and tertiary prevention.

5. Give examples of a person who is "at risk" for a health problem and factors that place the person at risk.

6. Differentiate among health, illness, and disease.

7. Identify the stages of disease and give an example of each stage.

8. Discuss the actions people take when they perceive that they are ill.

9. Describe the sick or dependent role.

10. Differentiate between independent and interdependent nursing actions.

III. Multiple choice

1. The major health problems in the United States today are:
- **a.** Chronic diseases and accidental injuries
- **b.** Of genetic origin
- **c.** Infectious diseases
- **d.** Occupational hazards

2. Screening for specific diseases is called:
- **a.** Primary prevention
- **b.** Rehabilitation
- **c.** Secondary prevention
- **d.** Altering risk factors

3. A syndrome is defined as:
- **a.** A disease of long duration
- **b.** The ultimate outcome of a disease
- **c.** The pattern of development of a disease
- **d.** A collection of signs and symptoms that indicate altered functioning

4. Healing that occurs with little treatment is called:
- **a.** Spontaneous resolution
- **b.** Miraculous healing
- **c.** Therapeutic intervention
- **d.** All of the above

5. The reasons for not seeking health care include which of the following?
- **a.** Fear of health care professionals or agencies
- **b.** Denial that symptoms are present
- **c.** Lack of knowledge concerning which symptoms require medical care
- **d.** All of the above

6. Which of the following factors affect health?
- **a.** Lead and arsenic
- **b.** High noise level
- **c.** Cold weather
- **d.** All of the above

7. A woman who perceives that certain symptoms indicate illness might display which behavior?
   a. Going to the health department
   b. Talking to a family member
   c. Waiting until she can afford medical assistance
   d. Selecting any of the above behaviors
8. A man who has recovered from a heart attack is expected to:
   a. Relinquish the sick role gradually
   b. Continue dependence
   c. Become independent immediately
   d. None of the above
9. The study of the cause of a disease is known as:
   a. The study of disease occurrence
   b. Etiology
   c. Evidence of a disease
   d. Medical interventions
10. Select the true statement from those listed below:
   a. Nursing interventions are directed toward restoring and maintaining optimal health.
   b. People who have signs and symptoms of illness always seek medical advice.
   c. The nursing actions based on analysis of specific data are called interdependent.
   d. Diseases are usually acute.

SUGGESTED READING

Tydell, P: Are there opportunities in your own backyard? Teaching health and self-care to the community, Nurs 87 17(6):77, 1987.

Chapter 2

Nursing Process: A Systematic Approach

JACQUELINE S. SPRAGUE

CHAPTER OBJECTIVES

On completion of this chapter, the student should be able to:

- Describe five steps of nursing process.
- Describe at least one framework that can be used for data collection and analysis.
- State four general conclusions that can be drawn from analysis of patient data.
- Define nursing diagnosis and describe the component parts.
- State five reasons for standardizing and classifying nursing diagnoses.
- Explain at least one method for setting priorities.
- Write goals in terms of observable patient behaviors.
- Describe five different action strategies for providing nursing care.
- Describe different methods of documentation.
- Identify the source of evaluation criteria.

PREREQUISITE READING

Long-Phipps, Chapter 2, pp. 11-23.

SELF-ASSESSMENT ACTIVITIES

I. Define the following terms.

Assessment	Nursing diagnosis
Baseline observation	Nursing process
Data analysis	Objective data
Evaluation criteria	Planning
Long-term goal	Problem-oriented record
NANDA	Subjective data
Nursing action	

II. Write your answers in the space provided.

1. What are the two most common frameworks used for nursing practice?

2. Why is it important to obtain assessment data by both the patient and the nurse?

3. What are four methods of data collection from specific sources?

4. Why is assessment data important?

5. What are the two primary components of a nursing diagnosis statement?

6. Why is a classification system of nursing diagnosis important?

7. Why should there be a mutual nurse-patient goal whenever possible?

8. What are the three criteria necessary for writing appropriate patient outcomes or goals?

9. What are five action strategies used by the nurse for providing nursing care?

10. Evaluation is based on which components of the nursing process?

11. What is the conceptual framework of your nursing program?

III. Multiple choice

1. The assessment process consists of:
   - **a.** Establishing goal-oriented actions
   - **b.** Determining desired patient outcomes to be achieved
   - **c.** Selecting action strategies to meet stated goals
   - **d.** Collecting data about the patient that is pertinent for providing nursing care
2. The best source of primary data about the patient is:
   - **a.** Significant others
   - **b.** The patient
   - **c.** The nurse
   - **d.** The physician
3. When analysis shows the patient is functioning inadequately, the nurse next:
   - **a.** Formulates a nursing goal
   - **b.** Makes a nursing diagnosis statement
   - **c.** Identifies nursing action
   - **d.** Reclassifies the data
4. A nursing diagnosis statement:
   - **a.** Is the diagnosis of the disease process
   - **b.** Is the treatment intervention for a disease process
   - **c.** Is the diagnosis and treatment of human responses to health problems
   - **d.** Refers to actual health problems, not potential health problems
5. Which statement about behavioral objectives is incorrect?
   - **a.** They provide criteria for evaluating patient progress.
   - **b.** They provide guidelines for determining nursing actions or interventions.
   - **c.** They indicate desired outcomes for the nurse.
   - **d.** They are derived from the nursing diagnosis.
6. The PES format refers to all of the following components of a nursing diagnosis except:
   - **a.** Medical diagnosis
   - **b.** Etiologic or related factors
   - **c.** The nursing diagnosis statement
   - **d.** Defining characteristics

7. Patient outcomes are written according to which of the following criteria?
   - a. Use verbs such as "understands" and "knows"
   - b. Do not include a time element
   - c. Serve as criteria for nursing diagnosis
   - d. Are stated as observable patient behaviors
8. Evaluation involves:
   - a. Comparing the actual outcome with the behavioral objective
   - b. Identifying and defining the problem
   - c. Establishing an initial plan of care
   - d. Formulating a hypothesis

IV. Label the terms below as either subjective data (S) or objective data (O).

_____ Decubitus 1 cm in diameter
_____ Headache
_____ Nausea
_____ Blood pressure reading
_____ X-ray report
_____ Diaphoresis
_____ Abdominal pain
_____ Depression
_____ Cyanosis
_____ Numbness

V. Listed below are the characteristics of the nursing process. Explain what each means.

1. Systematic
2. Purposeful
3. Interactional
4. Dynamic
5. Scientific

VI. Indicate which behavioral objective is stated correctly (C) and which is stated incorrectly (I).

1. _____ Patient will ambulate in A.M.
2. _____ Patient will consume one half of each meal served.
3. _____ Patient will know drugs.
4. _____ Patient will feel better.

CLINICAL ACTIVITY

Use an assessment form or nursing history form to collect data about an assigned patient in your clinical area. Analyze your findings and identify at least two problems of priority. Document these problems as a nursing diagnosis. Write goal statements, interventions, and evaluation criteria for each problem.

SUGGESTED READING

Reed, C: Patient care conferences: 3 fast steps to better patient care plans, Nurs 87, 17(3):66, 1987. How to improve patient care planning by planning ahead, including the patient, and observation.

Chapter 3

Nursing History and Physical Examination

JACQUELINE S. SPRAGUE

CHAPTER OBJECTIVES

On completion of this chapter the student should be able to:

- Describe ways to enhance a patient interview.
- Describe the purposes of a nursing history.
- Know where to find a sample nursing history and sample head-to-toe physical examination guide.
- Describe the four modalities for physical examination.
- Explain the basis for skin changes.
- Explain the differences between normal and abnormal lung sounds and heart sounds.
- Identify the parameters for describing lung and heart sounds
- Describe physical changes that may be observed during physical examination of the aged.

PREREQUISITE READING

Long-Phipps, Chapter 3, pp. 25-44.

SELF-ASSESSMENT ACTIVITIES

I. Define the following terms.

Adventitious breath sounds	PERRLA
Auscultation	Physical examination
Inspection	S_1 heart sound
Nursing history	S_2 heart sound
Palpation	Turgor
Percussion	Vesicular breath sounds

II. Write your answers in the space provided.

1. What are four guidelines for a successful patient interview?

2. What is the purpose of a nursing history?

3. Describe the four modalities of physical examination.

4. What is the most common approach used in performing a physical examination?

5. How would you initiate a patient interview for obtaining a nursing history? What would you say?

6. What are some of the more common physical assessment changes you would expect to see with aging?

III. Match each term with the appropriate definition.

1. _____	Macule	a.	Acne lesion
2. _____	Papule	b.	Erosion of skin surface
3. _____	Nodule	c.	Raised mass over 2 cm
4. _____	Tumor	d.	Freckle
5. _____	Vesicle	e.	Small blister
6. _____	Pustule	f.	Mole
7. _____	Ulcer	g.	Raised mass less than 1 cm

IV. Multiple choice

1. Skin pallor may be caused by:
   - a. Vasodilation
   - b. Deoxygenated hemoglobin
   - c. Increased bile pigment
   - d. Vasoconstriction
2. A patient's perception of his or her health problems is considered:
   - a. Subjective data
   - b. Objective data
3. The stethoscope is an effective tool used in which modality of physical examination?
   - a. Inspection
   - b. Auscultation
   - c. Palpation
   - d. Percussion
4. Vital skin signs are included in which area of nursing assessment?
   - a. Anterior chest
   - b. Extremities
   - c. General parameters
   - d. General survey
5. Cyanosis may be an indication of:
   - a. Edema
   - b. Vasospasm
   - c. Heart or lung disease
   - d. Liver disease
6. Having your patient follow your finger in an H configuration is a test for:
   - a. Corneal reflex
   - b. Visual acuity
   - c. Pupillary reflex
   - d. Extraocular movement
7. Tracheal deviation may indicate:
   - a. Pneumothorax
   - b. Pneumonia
   - c. Muscle weakness
   - d. Heart disease
8. Crackles or rales are caused by:
   - a. Rubbing of inflamed pleura between lung and chest wall
   - b. Air flowing through moisture in air passages
   - c. Air flowing through narrowed air passages
   - d. Closing of the mitral and tricuspid valves

9. The first heart sound (S_1) is heard best at:
   a. The base of the heart
   b. The third intercostal space
   c. The apex of the heart
   d. The second intercostal space

10. The second heart sound (S_2) is:
   a. The result of the closure of the aortic and pulmonic valves
   b. Heard best at the apex of the heart
   c. Located at the second intercostal space
   d. The result of the closing of the mitral and tricuspid valves

CLINICAL ACTIVITIES

1. Select a client in your clinical area. Using the form in your text, take a complete nursing history using good communication skills.
2. Perform a head and neck assessment according to the guide provided in text. Write a description of your findings and ask your clinical instructor to go over it with you.

SUGGESTED READING

McConnell, E: Getting the feel of lymph node assessment, 18(8):54, 1988.
Assessment techniques for the lymph node system using inspection and palpation. Excellent diagrams and example of important physical assessment technique. Includes head and neck assessment.

Chapter 4

Quality Assurance in Nursing

VIVIENNE I. WALTON

CHAPTER OBJECTIVES

On completion of this chapter, the student should be able to:

- Define quality assurance.
- Identify three reasons why quality assurance is an important aspect of the practice of nursing.
- Describe the steps of the American Nurses' Association (ANA) model of quality assurance.
- State the difference between standards and criteria.
- Name five mechanisms involved in implementing quality assurance programs.
- Describe the use of quality indicators as one means for monitoring quality of care.

PREREQUISITE READING

Long-Phipps, Chapter 4, pp. 45-55.

SELF-ASSESSMENT ACTIVITIES

I. Define the following terms.

Accountability
Aggregate data
Concurrent review (audit)
Criterion measure
DRG (diagnostic related groups)
Effectiveness
Efficiency
GNP (gross national product)
Incident reports
JCAH (Joint Commission on Accreditation of Hospitals)
Medical practice acts
Nurse practice acts
Nursing audit
Outcome criteria
Peer review
Process criteria
PSROs (professional standard review organizations)
Quality assurance
Quality assurance review committee
Quality indicators
Retrospective review (audit)
Standard
Standards of Nursing Practice
Structure criteria
Utilization review

II. Multiple choice

1. The primary function of the Professional Standards Review Organization (PSRO) is to:
   a. Evaluate competence of licensed health care professionals
   b. Develop standards for professional nursing practice
   c. Screen recipients of Medicaid funds
   d. Evaluate expenditures of federal monies for health care
2. The primary responsibility for implementing the standards of nursing practice lies with:
   a. The nursing director in the hospital
   b. Each individual nurse
   c. The nursing board within each state
   d. The physician writing the treatment orders
3. Which of the following defines the legal scope of nursing practice?
   a. Nurse practice acts
   b. Medical practice acts
   c. Joint Commission on Accreditation of Hospitals
   d. ANA *Standards of Nursing Practice*

4. JCAH (Joint Commission on Accreditation of Hospitals):
   a. Is a mandatory governmental program for accrediting hospitals
   b. Is a voluntary agency that licenses hospitals
   c. Establishes standards for the operation of hospitals
   d. Develops plans for monitoring the quality of nursing care
5. A quality assurance review program may focus on:
   a. The institution only
   b. The nurses and physicians only
   c. The care of the patients only
   d. The institution, the nurses, or patient care
6. A framework against which performance is compared is called:
   a. A criterion measure
   b. A standard
   c. Structure criterion
   d. Quality assurance
7. Criteria that will be used in the quality assurance evaluation process may be all of the following types *except:*
   a. Structure
   b. Process
   c. Assessment
   d. Outcome
8. The statement "Every patient will have oral hygiene as a part of the morning bath" is a(n):
   a. Assessment
   b. Standard
   c. Process criterion
   d. Outcome criterion
9. The statement "Intravenous infusions will be monitored every hour" is a(n):
   a. Process criterion
   b. Structure criterion
   c. Standard
   d. Outcome criterion
10. The statement "The patient can perform proper colostomy irrigations" is a(n):
    a. Process criterion
    b. Structure criterion
    c. Standard
    d. Outcome criterion
11. The statement "An RN will be available on every nursing unit" is a(n):
    a. Structure criterion
    b. Process criterion
    c. Outcome criterion
    d. Standard
12. The statement "The charge nurse on each shift will be an RN" is a(n):
    a. Standard
    b. Structure criterion
    c. Process criterion
    d. Outcome criterion
13. The Head Nurse (Nurse Manager) on the postsurgical unit asked the RN team leaders to randomly examine the nurse's notes on five of the preoperative patients on their team to see if preoperative teaching was done. This type of quality assurance review process is called:
    a. Retrospective
    b. Concurrent

14. The Head Nurse on an oncology unit wants to evaluate the quality of therapeutic communication used by her RN staff in caring for dying patients. Which type of monitoring system would be most appropriate?
    a. Nursing audit
    b. Peer review
    c. Patient satisfaction questionnaire
    d. Staff satisfaction questionnaire
15. Which are steps of the problem-solving model for the ANA's quality assurance process?
    a. Identify values, standards and criteria
    b. Measure degrees of attainment of standards and criteria, and interpret strengths and weaknesses
    c. Identify possible course of action, select, implement, and reevaluate action
    d. All of the above
16. Which is not considered a solution to an identified problem?
    a. Further clinical research into the problem
    b. Measurable assurance in terms of health
    c. Organization of peer pressure
    d. A reward system for improved compliance
17. Which may be considered a reason that a quality assurance review committee will need to focus more on ethical decision making in the future?
    a. Rapidly increasing opportunities in patient care, more options for patients and providers
    b. Continuance of diminished resources causing problems of distributive justice
    c. Participation of all health professionals in ethical decisions
    d. All of the above

III. For your consideration.

1. What effect do you think increased emphasis on cost containment has had upon the quality of health care?

2. What impact has the DRG reimbursement system had on nursing?

CLINICAL ACTIVITIES

1. Examine the quality assurance review process used within your clinical agency. What are the components? Compare the components used in your agency's review process with those identified in the ANA's model.
2. Attend a meeting of the quality assurance review committee for nursing in your agency. How does the committee decide what to focus their review on? How often does the membership of the committee change? How does one become a member of the committee? How is confidentiality maintained in the review process? What type of review process is utilized-retrospective or concurrent? Does the committee ever focus on any ethical issues in the review process?
3. Talk with the Nurse Manager (Head Nurse) on your assigned clinical unit to find out what stengths and weaknesses have been identified for the unit as a result of a quality assurance review evaluation. What course of action has been planned to reduce or eliminate weaknesses and reinforce strengths?

SUGGESTED READINGS

Hack, KB: Where is quality assurance going? . . .nurse profile, J Nurs Adm 18(5):33, 1988.

Hamilton, S and others: Unit level quality assurance: essential for sources, Rehabil Nurs 13(2):76-78, 92, 1988.

Harrington, P and others: Standards and quality assurance—a common sense approach. . .unit-based quality assurance, Nurs Manage 19(1):24-27, 1988.

Kanar, RJ: The influence of a quality assurance program on patient satisfaction. J Nurs Qual Assur 2(3):18-24, 1988.

Kibbee, P: An emerging program: the quality assurance nurse, J Nurs Adm 18(4):30-33, 1988.

Latreille, DD and others: Quality assurance, J Pediatr Nurs 2(5):291-294, 1987.

McCourt, AE: Implementation of nursing diagnosis through integration with quality assurance, Nurs Clin North Am 22(4):899-904, 1987.

Osinski, E: Developing patient outcomes as a quality measure of nursing care, Nurs Manage 18(10):28-29, 1987.

Pearlson, JG: Development and implementation of systematic monitoring of medication errors, J Nurs Qual Assur 2(2):77-81, 1988.

Puetz, B: Evaluation of quality assurance in nursing care, Rehabil Nurs 13(2):64, 1988.
Suila, L and others: Quality assurance . . . ask the patient, Nurs Time 83(45):40-42, 1987.
Sutton, LD and others: Computerized data bases: an integrated approach to monitoring quality of patient care, Arch Phys Med Rehabil 68(2):850-853, 1988.

UNIT II Health Promotion

Chapter 5

Developmental Factors Affecting Health of Adults

BRENDA GOODNER

CHAPTER OBJECTIVES

On completion of this chapter, the student should be able to:

- Describe physical development characteristics of each adult age group.
- Describe changes in sexuality characteristics of each adult age group.
- Describe the characteristics of the three adult stages of psychologic development.
- Describe the developmental tasks of young, middle, and late adulthood.
- Identify the health needs of each adult age group.
- Identify the major health concerns of each adult age group.
- Describe general nursing interventions for the elderly patient.

PREREQUISITE READING

Long-Phipps, Chapter 5, pp. 59-75.

SELF-ASSESSMENT ACTIVITIES

I. Define the following terms.

Activity theory
Alzheimer's disease
Chronic dementia
Development
Disengagement theory
Generativity versus stagnation
Growth
Integrity versus despair
Intimacy versus isolation
Presbyopia

II. Write your answers in the space provided.

1. List the six major tasks of young adulthood.

2. List the tasks of late adulthood.

3. Discuss the adult development stage of intimacy versus isolation and its resolution.

4. Discuss the stage of generativity versus stagnation and its resolution.

III. Multiple choice

1. The stage at which an individual begins to take stock of his or her life and to assess potential for the future is:
   a. Integrity versus despair
   b. Industry versus inferiority
   c. Generativity versus stagnation
   d. Functional versus dysfunctional
2. Patterns of physical and psychosocial development in our society are:
   a. Varied
   b. Continuous
   c. Structured
   d. Predictable
3. Research indicates that the most significant contributing factor to enjoyable sexual relations for a person aged 45 to 69 is:
   a. Physical capacity to perform
   b. Previous sexual satisfaction
   c. Satisfaction with partner
   d. Prevailing cultural attitudes
4. The priority goal of nursing care of the older person is:
   a. Pain relief
   b. Prevention of illness
   c. Optimal functioning
   d. Rehabilitation
5. The planning phase of the nursing process emphasizes which theoretical framework in determining goals for the elderly patient?
   a. Prevention
   b. Environment
   c. Self-care
   d. Dependence
6. Metabolism of drugs in the elderly can be altered as lower levels of enzyme activity occurs. Which major organ is involved?
   a. Brain
   b. Liver
   c. Intestines
   d. Pancreas
7. The elderly are at higher risk of suffering toxic levels of medications routinely. This is related to:
   a. Decreased renal clearance
   b. Decreased liver functioning
   c. Decreased congnitive functioning
   d. Generally decreased circulation

8. In analyzing care of the elderly, which nursing diagnosis should be most prominently considered?
   a. Fear of death
   b. Sympathy
   c. Independence
   d. Powerlessness
9. Which of the following activities would help a 70-year-old woman maintain self-worth and independence?
   a. Call her "Grandma" so she'll feel at home.
   b. Speak loudly to be sure she hears you.
   c. Give her a bath to conserve her energy.
   d. Give her as much control as possible.
10. One of the developmental tasks of middle adulthood is:
   a. Developing a sense of social responsibility
   b. Adjusting to declining physical strength
   c. Reevaluating life's goals
   d. Forming a meaningful philosophy of life
11. What is the age-related pattern for interest in sexual activity?
   a. Diminishes in middle adulthood
   b. Diminishes after menopause
   c. Is absent in late adulthood
   d. May continue into the 80s and 90s
12. Which of the following philosophical views would be most appropriate for the nurse to have when working with the elderly?
   a. Aging is a period of approaching death.
   b. Aging is a time for withdrawing from life to make room for younger persons.
   c. Aging is an inevitable process requiring adaptations in living patterns.
   c. Aging is a process that persons should do everything possible to delay.
13. The major problem that the elderly patient is prone to develop because of alterations in the distribution, metabolism, and excretion of drugs is:
   a. Toxicity
   b. Gastrointestinal distress
   c. Fluid overload
   d. Stroke
14. The primary health concerns of young adults are directly related to:
   a. Fears of growing old
   b. Social isolation
   c. Fears of declining sexual functioning
   d. Stresses of social and career achievements
15. The conflict of middle adulthood is:
   a. Intimacy versus isolation
   b. Generativity versus stagnation
   c. Integrity versus despair
   d. Industry versus shame and doubt
16. To promote sleep in the elderly, the nurse should first:
   a. Use independent measures, such as a back rub or bedtime snack
   b. Explain to the patient the importance of sleep
   c. Administer a prescribed sedative
   d. Identify factors that are disturbing sleep

IV. What are the major physiologic changes of aging in each major system of the body?

1. Cardiovascular system

2. Respiratory system

3. Nervous system

4. Musculoskeletal system

5. Gastrointestinal system

6. Urinary system

SUGGESTED READINGS

Burggraf, V and Donlon, B: Assessing the elderly (Part 1), Am J Nurs 85:974-984, Sept 1985.
Overview of techniques used for physical examination. Provided is a chart that describes the problems of aging occurring in each body system, factors causing the problem, conditions that should be ruled out, and what to teach the patient/family about the problem.

Hahn, AB and others: Mosby's pharmacology in nursing, St. Louis, 1985, The CV Mosby Co.

Henderson, ML: Assessing the elderly: a two-part CE feature. Part Two: Altered Presentations, Am J Nurs 85:1103-1106, Oct 1985.

Chapter 6

Health Promotion: Nutrition and Exercise

MARY S. NICHOLS

CHAPTER OBJECTIVES

On completion of this chapter, the student should be able to:

- Describe factors affecting health-promoting behaviors.
- Identify the major nutrients required for body needs.
- Describe the interrelationships between food and drugs.
- Use the daily food guide to evaluate adequacy of nutrient intake.
- Define obesity and identify medical and nursing interventions to facilitate weight loss.
- Define underweight and identify interventions to facilitate weight gain.
- Discuss difficulties that may occur with tube feedings or total parenteral nutrition.
- Describe the effects and benefits of exercise.
- Describe recommendations for physical fitness programs.
- Differentiate between isometric and isotonic exercises.

PREREQUISITE READING

Long-Phipps, Chapter 6, pp. 77-96.

SELF-ASSESSMENT ACTIVITIES

I. Define the following terms.

Activity tolerance assessment
Aerobic exercise
Anorexia
Fad diets
Fasting diets
Gastric positioning
Health promotion
Horizontal stapling
Hyperplastic hypertrophia
Intestinal bypass
Isometric exercise
Isotonic exercise
Lactovegetarian
Morbid obesity
Protein calorie malnutrition
TPN
Valsalva maneuver
Vegan diet
Vertical stapling

II. Comment on each phase of behavior modification for changing the pattern of eating and exercising.

1. Setting own goals

2. Self-monitoring

3. Developing a personal reward system

4. Obtaining positive feedback

5. Developing a new self-concept of thinness

6. Developing and implementing an activity program

III. **A.** List six criteria for bypass surgery.

B. Complete the following table.

Therapeutic modality	Description	Postoperative highlights
Bypass surgery		
Gastric partitioning		
Intestinal bypass		
Gastric balloon		

IV. Briefly explain the following concepts.

1. Factors affecting health-promotion behaviors

2. Nutrients needed throughout life

3. Nutrient needs are affected by

4. The most common nutritional alterations are

5. Obese persons are at risk for

6. Medications may affect nutritional status

7. Methods of weight reduction are

8. The effect of behavior modification on an obese person's weight reduction program

9. Exercise has a positive effect on body systems

V. Multiple choice

Mr. Reynaud is postoperative from a cholecystectomy. The nurse is preparing to assist him with his preparations for discharge. His physician has prescribed a 1000-calorie diet until his next office visit, which is scheduled in 3 weeks.

1. Which of the following statements should *not* be included in the nurse's instructions?
   a. Changes in eating patterns are usually required for permanent weight loss.
   b. Rapid weight loss is usually the result of loss of fluid rather than fat.
   c. Protein intake should be maintained.
   d. A salt-free diet should be recommended.
2. Mrs. Raynaud said to the nurse, "My husband likes to eat a bedtime snack. What should he eat at night?" The correct response to her question is:
   a. "Skim milk, 1/2 glass, and a graham cracker."
   b. "One-half turkey sandwich and a glass of milk."
   c. "A small box of raisins."
   d. "Let's look at the dietician's recommendations on the diet sheet."
3. Mr. Raynaud tells his nurse that his brother is also very obese and requests her recommendations for helping his brother lose weight. The nurse's best reply is:
   a. "You are concerned about your brother's problem?"
   b. "Advise him to make an appointment with his physician."
   c. "Your brother should increase his daily exercise to promote weight loss."
   d. "He's genetically predisposed to obesity and will need behavior modification."
4. For a patient recovering from gastric partitioning, the feedings should begin with:
   a. Pureed food
   b. Vitamin supplements
   c. Clear fluids
   d. Soft blend foods
5. The gastric balloon is a temporary measure to facilitate weight loss. Postprocedure instructions should include all *except:*
   a. Diet should progress to 1000 calories
   b. Antacids every 2 hours
   c. Avoid coffee, alcohol and tobacco
   d. Participate in an exercise program
6. Sally is 26 years old and is 25% underweight. Her main complaint is lack of appetite. The nurse who is doing a nutritional assessment should ask:
   a. "Do you fail to eat when you are hungry?"
   b. "Why don't you like to eat?"
   c. "Have you ever had mental problems?"
   d. "How many calories do you eat each day?"

Mr. Gonya is being discharged from the hospital with medical orders for home therapy of TPN. His discharge summary should include instruction about prevention of infection.

7. Mr. Gonya's wife should be instructed to change the dressing of the operative site:
   a. Daily
   b. Every 2 to 3 days each week
   c. Once every 2 weeks
   d. Once a week
8. Mrs. Gonya should be instructed concerning the infusion rate and signs of:
   a. Hypoglycemia
   b. Overhydration
   c. Hyperglycemia
   d. All of the above
9. Mr. Gonya has cirrhosis of the liver; therefore, his diet should be:
   a. High in protein
   b. Low in carbohydrates
   c. Moderate in protein
   d. High fat

10. For a person who is receiving bolus delivery of tube feeding, the nurse should:
    a. Set the pump rate for 3-hours delivery time
    b. Infuse 300-400 ml in a few minutes
    c. Dilute the tube feeding
    d. Place the crushed and dissolved medication in the feeding tube
11. Persons receiving TPN should also be monitored for:
    a. Sugar and acetone in urine
    b. Maintenance of weight
    c. Electrolyte or fluid imbalance
    d. All of the above

Mr. Radner's cardiologist has prescribed aerobic exercise as part of his recovery program. Mr. Radner asks the nurse to describe the benefits of this type of exercise.

12. The most appropriate response for the nurse is:
    a. "It will help control your weight."
    b. "It will help you sleep."
    c. "What did your doctor tell you?"
    d. "Aerobic exercise will help you stop smoking and drinking."
13. Mr. Radner asks the nurse how aerobics will help his circulatory system. The best reply is:
    a. "Aerobic exercise helps your blood return to the heart."
    b. "It lowers your blood pressure."
    c. "Aerobics is good for your heart."
    d. "Aerobics maintains endurance."
14. Mr. Radner tells his nurse that his favorite form of exercise is playing baseball with his children and his neighbors. Baseball is:
    a. An aerobic exercise
    b. An anaerobic exercise
15. The target pulse of a person recovering from myocardial infarction would probably be prescribed at:
    a. 50% to 60% maximum heart rate
    b. 70% to 85% of maximum heart rate
    c. Baseline level plus five beats
    d. Baseline level of 25 beats

CLINICAL ACTIVITIES

1. Write a teaching plan for a patient who is preparing for discharge. The patient will manage his own TPN. See the guidelines for TPN in Chapter 3 text, pp. 89-91.

2. Write another teaching plan for a patient going home with a gastric balloon or tube feeding.

SUGGESTED READINGS

Blessing, DL, and others: The physiologic effects of eight weeks of aerobic dance, with and without hand-held weights, Am J Sports Med 15(5):508-510, 1988.

Gwinup, G: Weight loss without dietary restriction: efficacy of different forms of aerobic exercise, Am J Sports Med 15(3):275-279, 1987.
Interesting results comparing weight loss without dietary restrictions.

Morrisey, MJ: Exercise and chronic heart disease, Geriatr Nurs 8(3), 1987.
Discusses health promotion of aging person. Assessment, prescription, exercise session, references.

Safran, MR, and others: The role of warm-ups in muscular injury prevention, Am J Sports Med 16(2):123-127, 1988.

UNIT III Common Problems Encountered in Medical-Surgical Nursing

Chapter 7

Stress and Stress Management

VIVIENNE I. WALTON

CHAPTER OBJECTIVES

On completion of this chapter, the student should be able to:

- Differentiate between stress and stressor, and explain the relationship of stress to optimal functioning and growth.
- Identify factors influencing stress response.
- Describe physiologic and behavioral responses to stress.
- Define coping and describe types of coping strategies.
- Identify assessment parameters of and interventions for anxiety.
- Describe the nature of crisis and approach to crisis intervention.
- Describe methods of stress management.

PREREQUISITE READING

Long-Phipps, Chapter 7, pp. 99-115.

Study thoroughly

1. Defense mechanisms
2. Levels of anxiety
3. Stages of crisis

SELF-ASSESSMENT ACTIVITIES

I. Define the following terms.

Adaptation
Adrenocorticotropic (ACTH)
Alarm reaction stage
Anterior pituitary-adrenocortical mechanism
Autogenic training
Benson's relaxation response
Biofeedback
Coping
Corticotropin-releasing factor (CRF)
Eustress
Exhaustion stage
General adaptation syndrome (GAS)
Local adaptation syndrome (LAS)
Maladaptation
Medulla
Perception
Progressive relaxation
Resistance stage
Situational crisis
Stress
Stressors
Sympathetic adrenal medullary
Therapeutic groups
Unified whole

II. Multiple choice

1. Which of the following is psychologic adaptation–directed?
   - **a.** Self-esteem
   - **b.** Eustress
   - **c.** Preservation of self-identity and self-esteem
   - **d.** Self-concept
2. Which of the following is the general adaptation syndrome (GAS) proposed by Selye as a response of individuals to stress?
   - **a.** Alarm reaction
   - **b.** Resistance
   - **c.** Exhaustion
   - **d.** All of the above
3. Which of the following response to stress is influenced by the stimulus characteristics?
   - **a.** Intensity
   - **b.** Duration
   - **c.** Number
   - **d.** All of the above
4. Which of the following is not considered to be a stress management therapy?
   - **a.** Biofeedback
   - **b.** Health promotion
   - **c.** Behavioral change programs
   - **d.** Systematic desensitization
5. Behavioral reactions to stress include which of the following?
   - **a.** Anxiety and aggressiveness
   - **b.** Depression and withdrawal
   - **c.** Suspicion and somatization
   - **d.** All of the above
6. There are many types of coping strategies. Which is not identified as a type?
   - **a.** Action, cognitive
   - **b.** Interpsychic, impersonal
   - **c.** Emotional
   - **d.** Intrapsychic, interpersonal
7. Which are the two defense mechanisms that are frequently manifested by the hospitalized patient?
   - **a.** Projection and rejection
   - **b.** Denial and repression
   - **c.** Suppression and displacement
   - **d.** Identification and conversion
8. The Shontz's phases of crisis are all of the following except:
   - **a.** Initial impact, realization
   - **b.** Defense retreat, acknowledgment
   - **c.** Adaptation
   - **d.** Denial, acceptance

III. Fill in the blanks.

a. Antianxiety
b. Benzodiazepines
c. Crisis
d. Depressants
e. Epinephrine
f. Norepinephrine
g. Relaxation
h. Unconscious
i. Therapeutic

1. _____ occurs when anxiety overwhelms the self and the person is unable to use coping mechanisms.
2. The most frequently prescribed antianxiety agents are the _____.
3. Alcohol or other CNS _____ should be avoided when taking _____ agents.
4. _____ is the opposite of tension produced by stress.

Continued

5. Defense mechanisms are _____ mechanisms used by individuals in adjustment to life stress.
6. _____ groups consist of persons who are experiencing common stressors.
7. The sympathetic-adrenal medullary response prepares the person for "fight or flight" through release of _____ and _____.

CASE STUDY

Carol Linley, a 31-year-old RN, arrived home from work to find her neighbor, Sharon, at her doorstep. Sharon was extremely tense as she announced the news about Carol's husband, Len. "I've got some terrible news. Len's been in an automobile accident. He's now at St. Thomas Hospital emergency room," said Sharon nervously. "Oh my God, I must go to him. Sharon, please watch the children for me," cried Carol as she dashed into the house to call her father-in-law, who was retired and at home most of the time.

When Carol and her father-in-law arrived at the hospital, the doctor greeted them and informed them that Len had died from massive hemorrhage secondary to multiple injuries.

The emergency room was a mad house. The woman whose car had hit Len's car was crying out hysterically. There were several other persons being treated for injuries and moaning loudly. Despite the high noise level, Carol looked at her father-in-law with a calm, blank look on her face, took his hand and said, "Come, we must let Mom (her mother-in-law) know."

When Carol and her in-laws arrived back at her house, Sharon met them and informed Carol that her two children had been put to bed at her house. Carol was walking around as if she were in a daze. She began to busy herself with housework while some of her close friends and neighbors visited.

At one point, while preparing tea in the kitchen, a few tears came to Carol's eyes. She asked a friend to have a doctor prescribe a tranquilizer for her so that she could deal with the grief of Len's death. She felt frozen, unbelieving, and resolved that she would not cry. Her in-laws stayed with her that night.

The next morning, Carol called her parents, Len's employer, a funeral director, and the family lawyer. When the children came home later that morning, she sat them down and told them of their father's death. She embraced them as they cried and said, "We're going to make it."

1. Where do you perceive stress, adaptation, and coping in the above situation?
2. Where do you detect ineffective coping?
3. What type of crisis created adaptive demands for Carol?
4. What action-focused coping strategies did Carol demonstrate?
5. What emotion-focused coping strategies did Carol demonstrate?

SUGGESTED READINGS

Booth, DM, and others: Nursing process: stress in nursing school, AD Nurse 32(2):29-30, 1988.
Curtin, LL: Coping with stress, Nurs Manage 19(6):7, 1988.
Fletcher, J: Stress management, Intensive Care Nurse 3(2):56-60, 1987.
Gillespie, C: Stress-reducing strategies, Nurs Time 83(39):30-32, 1987.
Gorton, D: Holistic health techniques to increase individual coping and wellness, Perioper Nurse Q 3(3):41-50, 1987.
Howden, C: Coping with stress—sharing and learning, Senior Nurs 7(2):6-8, 1987.
Hradek, EA: Crisis intervention and suicide, J Psychosoc Nurs Ment Health Serv 26(5):24, 25 27, 1988.
Jones, LH: How to assess stress: a significant step for the nursing student . . . factors that impact on the health of students, J Nurs Educ 27(5):227-228, 1988.
Knapp, TR: Stress versus strain: a methodological critique, Nurs Res 37(3):181-184, 1988.
Moch, SD: Towards a personal control/uncontrol balance, J Adv Nurs 13(1):119-123, 1988.
Wheeler, BR: Crisis intervention: recognizing and helping patients overcome anxiety, J Adm OR Nurs 47(5):1242, 1244, 1248, 1988.

Chapter 8

Fluid and Electrolyte Imbalances

MARY S. NICHOLS

CHAPTER OBJECTIVES

On completion of this chapter, the student should be able to:

- Describe the mechanisms for maintaining fluid and electrolyte balance.
- Describe the mechanisms and effects of fluid deficit and excess.
- Describe the mechanisms and effects of deficits and excesses of sodium, potassium, calcium, and magnesium.
- Describe the mechanisms that maintain acid-base balance.
- Differentiate among metabolic and respiratory acidosis and alkalosis, and describe the causes and effects of each type.
- Identify data indicating fluid or electrolyte imbalances.
- Describe the management of patients with fluid and electrolyte imbalances.

PREREQUISITE READING

Long-Phipps, Chapter 8, pp. 117-141.

SELF-ASSESSMENT ACTIVITIES

I. Define the following terms.

Acidosis
Aldosterone
Alkalosis
Antidiuretic hormone
Bicarbonate
Buffer
Carbon dioxide narcosis
Carbonic acid
Chvostek's sign
Dehydration
Diffusion
Edema
Electrolyte
Filtration
Hypercalcemia
Hyperkalemia
Hypermagnesemia
Hypernatremia
Hyperpotassemia
Hypertonic
Hypocalcemia
Hypokalemia
Hypomagnesemia
Hypopotassemia
Hypotonic
Ions
Isotonic
Ketoacidosis
Metabolic acidosis
Metabolic alkalosis
Oncotic pressure
Osmolality
Osmosis
Osmotic diuresis
Osmotic pressure
Overhydration
Parathormone
Potential fluid spaces
Respiratory acidosis
Respiratory alkalosis
Solutes
Solvent
Starling's law of the capillaries
Tetany
Third spacing of fluids
Tonicity
Trousseau's sign
Water intoxication

II. Write the answer to the following questions in the space provided.

1. List four factors at the arteriole end of the capillary that affect hydrostatic pressure.

2. List the primary factor and three secondary factors at the venule end of the capillary that affect hydrostatic pressure.
Primary:

Secondary:

3. List the primary factor and three secondary factors that affect colloid osmotic pressure.
Primary:

Secondary:

4. List three physiologic mechanisms that can lead to edema.

III. Identify the acid-base imbalance for each of the arterial blood gas reports below. Also, indicate whether there is compensation and explain the mechanism of compensation. What would be the treatment for each of the imbalances?

		Normal
1.	pH = 7.20	pH = 7.35 to 7.45
	PCO^2 = 50	PCO^2 = 38 to 42 mm Hg
	HCO^3 = 28	HCO^3 = 23 to 25 mEq/L
2.	pH = 7.50	
	PCO^2 = 38	
	HCO^3 = 30	
3.	pH = 7.18	
	PCO^2 = 37	
	HCO^3 = 16	

IV. Briefly discuss the following concepts.

1. Explain the meaning of the following statement:

No single electrolyte can be out of balance without causing fluid and other electrolytes to be out of balance also.

2. How does potassium help to maintain acid-base balance?

3. Why are elderly patients more at risk for fluid imbalances than younger adult patients?

V. Test your assessment skills.

An elderly male was transferred to the hospital from a nursing home with a diagnosis of malnutrition and dehydration. His serum electrolyte report showed the following:

Sodium 155 (135 to 145 mEq/L)
Potassium 2.0 (3.5 to 4.5 mEq/L)
Chloride 80 (90 to 110 mEq/L)
Bicarbonate 18 (24 to 28)
Magnesium 4.7 (1.5 to 2.5)

1. What acid-base imbalance is the patient experiencing?

2. Because of the type of acid-base imbalance that exists in the patient, what clinical manifestations would you anticipate finding upon assessing the patient? List them.

3. What type of sodium, potassium, and magnesium imbalance is the patient experiencing?

4. Because of the type of sodium imbalance that exists in the patient, what clinical manifestations would you anticipate finding upon assessing the patient? List them.

5. Because of the type of potassium imbalance that exists in the patient, what clinical manifestations would you anticipate finding upon assessing the patient? List them.

6. What clinical manifestations would you expect to find because of the type of magnesium imbalance that exists in the patient? List them.

VI. Multiple choice

1. The most common manifestations of hyposmolar imbalance are caused by:
   a. Osmotic diuresis
   b. Severe deficit in serum calcium
   c. Swelling of the brain cells
   d. Excess intravascular fluid loss
2. A hyperosmolar imbalance is manifested by:
   a. Edema
   b. Weight gain
   c. Low serum sodium
   d. Dehydration
3. The most prominent clinical manifestations of extracellular fluid volume deficit are:
   a. Postural hypotension and tachycardia
   b. Dry mucous membranes and dry skin
   c. Decreased urinary output and edema
   d. Poor skin turgor and headache
4. The most prominent sign of extracellular fluid volume excess is:
   a. Edema
   b. Postural hypotension
   c. Increased urinary output
   d. Weight loss

5. The best indicator of fluid volume status is:
   a. Measurement of intake and output
   b. Blood pressure
   c. Daily weight
   d. Activity level
6. The clinical finding that is not characteristic of acidosis (both respiratory and metabolic) is:
   a. Excess hydrogen ion concentration
   b. Hyperventilation
   c. Hyperkalemia
   d. Tetany
7. The clinical finding that is not characteristic of alkalosis (both metabolic and respiratory) is:
   a. Hypokalemia
   b. Arterial blood pH below normal levels
   c. Numbness and tingling of fingers and toes
   d. Hypokalemia
8. Respiratory alkalosis can be caused by any condition that causes the patient to:
   a. Vomit excessively
   b. Hyperventilate
   c. Have diarrhea
   d. Develop an obstruction of the airway
9. Metabolic acidosis is a common problem with all of the following conditions *except*:
   a. Salicylate intoxication
   b. Renal failure
   c. Chronic obstructive lung disease
   d. Diarrhea
10. Metabolic alkalosis will not occur with which of the following interventions?
    a. Reducing dietary intake of sodium
    b. Keeping edematous extremities in a dependent position
    c. Administering diuretics
    d. Restricting fluid intake
11. Which of the following is *not* a treatment for edema?
    a. Reducing dietary intake of sodium
    b. Keeping edematous extremities in a dependent position
    c. Administering diuretics
    d. Restricting fluid intake
12. Kayexalate is used to treat:
    a. Hyperkalemia
    b. Hypercalcemia
    c. Hypermagnesemia
    d. Hypernatremia
13. Trousseau's sign and Chvostek's sign are done to assess for:
    a. Hypocalcemia
    b. Hypokalemia
    c. Hypomagnesemia
    d. Hyponatremia
14. Which of the following is *not* recommended for the prevention of osteoporosis?
    a. Stop smoking
    b. Take calcium supplements with vitamin D
    c. Exercise regularly
    d. Reduce the intake of oysters and other shellfish
15. The primary treatment for hypernatremia that occurs without water excess is:
    a. Performing a gastric washing
    b. Administering potassium chloride
    c. Encouraging a liberal intake of water
    d. Restricting fluid intake

16. Insensible fluid loss occurs through all of the following routes *except:*
   a. Skin
   b. Kidneys
   c. Lungs
   d. Gastrointestinal tract

VII. Match the fluid volume imbalances below with the appropriate situation.

a. Hypertonic **c.** ECF volume excess
b. Hypotonic **d.** ECF volume deficit

1. ______ A comatose patient receiving tube feedings via a nasogastric tube
2. ______ A patient who consumes a diet of green leafy vegetables and lots of water
3. ______ A patient who has chronic profuse drainage from an intestinal fistula
4. ______ A patient who ingests a large quantity of glucose
5. ______ A patient who has a decreased cardiac output and decreased venous return secondary to congestive heart failure
6. ______ A person whose kidney function is diminished and ingests large amounts of water
7. ______ A patient who is hemorrhaging
8. ______ A patient who receives multiple tap water enemas
9. ______ An elderly person who drinks only one glass of liquids per day
10. ______ A person who has prolonged vomiting and diarrhea
11. ______ A patient who has excessive drainage and protein loss from a massive third-degree burn

VIII. Complete the chart below. Then underline the most prominent clinical findings with each imbalance.

	Hypocalcemia	Hypomagnesemia
Causes		
Clinical findings		
Causes		
Clinical findings		

IX. Multiple choice

1. The minimum daily requirement for sodium is:
   a. 1 g c. 3 g
   b. 2 g d. 4 g

2. Which food would be best for a patient with hypokalemia?
   a. Well-cooked squash
   b. Raw cantaloupe
   c. Boiled peanuts
   d. Liver
3. Which of the following is not a buffer system of the body?
   a. Proteins
   b. Carbonic acid-bicarbonate
   c. Phosphates
   d. Carbohydrates
4. If the nurse detects that a patient receiving an intravenous infusion of 5% dextrose in water is developing fluid overload, the nurse should do all of the following *except*:
   a. Discontinue the infusion immediately
   b. Notify the physician
   c. Decrease flow rate
   d. Check the patient's output
5. When hydrostatic pressure in the arteriole end of the blood vessel is greater than the colloid osmotic pressure in the capillary bed, fluid will:
   a. Move from the interstitial space to the vascular space
   b. Move from the vascular space to the interstitial space
   c. Remain in the vascular space, thus causing symptoms of fluid overload
   d. Be excreted from the kidney at a more rapid rate
6. In the adult male, water makes up 60% of body weight, whereas in the adult female, water makes up only 50% of body weight. The primary reason for this difference in body fluid is that:
   a. Women contain more body fat than men
   b. Men normally drink more water than women
   c. Women perspire more than men
   d. Men consume more salt in their diets than women
7. Electrolytes perform all of the following functions *except*:
   a. Promote neuromuscular irritability
   b. Regulate acid-base balance
   c. Maintain proper functioning of the GI tract
   d. Maintain body fluid volume and osmolality
8. Marian Clouser's serum calcium level is 3.0 (normal is 4.5 to 5.8 mEq/L). The nurse also detects that Marian has a positive Chovstek's sign. To document a positive Chovstek's sign, the nurse would chart which of the following?
   a. Palmar flexion of the hand when circulation is restricted for a few seconds by grasping the wrist
   b. Sluggish deep patellar reflexes
   c. Poor skin turgor and slow capillary refill
   d. Twitching of the facial muscles when the facial nerve tapped just below the temporal area
9. The primary stimulus controlling fluid intake is:
   a. Serum sodium level
   b. Thirst
   c. Urinary output
   d. Body weight
10. For calcium to be absorbed from the GI tract, which of the following must also be present?
   a. Calcitonin
   b. Vitamin D
   c. Potassium
   d. Glucose
11. To maintain a stable pH, the bicarbonate to carbonic acid ratio must be maintained at:
   a. 20:1
   b. 1:20
   c. 2:1
   d. 1:2

12. Hypernatremia and hyperosmolar imbalance are similar in that:
    a. With both imbalances the primary problem is a significant decrease in water in relation to solute (mainly sodium) concentration
    b. With both there is an increase in both water and sodium proportionately
    c. With both there is a significant decrease in water and sodium proportionately
    d. With both there is a significant decrease in solutes (mainly sodium) concentration in relation to water
13. A patient's serum potassium level is 7.0 (normal is 3.5 to 5.5 mEq/L). When making additional assessments of the patient, the nurse would expect to find all of the follwing *except*:
    a. Tall, peaked T-waves on the ECG tracing
    b. Hyperreflexia
    c. Skeletal muscle spasms
    d. Diarrhea
14. When an acid-base imbalance occurs, in which order will the mechanisms regulating acid-base balance respond?
    a. Chemical buffers, kidneys, respiratory system
    b. Respiratory system, kidneys, chemical buffers
    c. Kidneys, chemical buffers, respiratory system
    d. Chemical buffers, respiratory system, kidneys

X. For each of the fluid compartments below, place the electrolytes in the compartment in which it is most abundant.

$HPO_4^=$	Mg^{++}	HCO_3
Ca^{++}	K^+	$SO_4^=$
Cl^-	$Prot^-$	NA^+

Extracellular **Intracellular**

2. What is the most abundant extracellular anion?

3. What is the most abundant intracellular anion?

4. What is the most abundant extracellular cation?

5. What is the most abundant intracellular cation?

CLINICAL ACTIVITIES

1. Assess your next patient in the clinical area for manifestations of a fluid, electrolyte, and/or acid-base imbalance. Don't forget to check results of laboratory reports such as ECG, arterial blood gases (if performed), serum electrolytes, and urinalysis (for specific gravity).

SUGGESTED READINGS

Beil, AV: Osteoporosis: how to avoid its crippling effect, RN 49:14-47, Aug 1986.
Identifies high-risk patients and causes. Describes how to reduce the odds of developing osteoporosis, problems that occur as a result of osteoporosis, and how it's diagnosed.

Elbaum, N: With cancer patients, be alert for hypercalcemia, Nursing 14:58-59, Aug 1984.
Through a case study, the author describes how hypercalcemia develops in cancer patients, the signs and symptoms, what to do to treat it, and how to prevent it.

Folk-Lighty, M: Solving the puzzles of patients with fluid imbalance, Nursing 14:34-41, Feb 1984.
The author uses four different case studies to describe parameters for assessing fluid imbalance, mechanisms involved in body fluid regulation, four types of fluid volume imbalances, and sodium imbalances.

RN Master care plan: preventing electrolyte imbalances, RN 47:32-34, Nov 1984.
A standard care plan that outlines nursing diagnoses, goals, and interventions for patients with fluid volume imbalances, and potassium, sodium, and calcium imbalances.

Stark, JL and Hunt, V: Managing fluid and electrolyte imbalances, Nursing 14:56G, 57, 56N, 56R, July 1984.
Describes the causes, signs and symptoms, and treatments for fluid volume excesses and deficits, and potassium, sodium, phosphate, and magnesium imbalances.

Williams, SR: Water and electrolytes. In Nutrition and diet therapy, St. Louis, 1985, The CV Mosby Co.

Chapter 9

Shock

MARY S. NICHOLS

CHAPTER OBJECTIVES

On completion of this chapter, the student should be able to:

- Contrast three major types of shock.
- Describe early and late pathophysiologic changes that occur with shock.
- Describe organ damage that may occur with shock.
- Describe different methods of monitoring for shock.
- Describe methods of fluid replacement during shock.
- Identify effects of pharmacologic agents used to treat shock and nursing measures for patients receiving drug therapy.
- Describe therapeutic measures for shock other than fluids and drug therapy.

PREREQUISITE READING

Long-Phipps, Chapter 9, pp. 143-166.

SELF-ASSESSMENT ACTIVITIES

I. Match the chemicals below with the appropriate description.

a. Aldosterone **c.** Renin
b. Histamine **d.** Lactic acid

1. _____ Secreted by the juxtaglomerular cells
2. _____ Causes sodium and water retention in the kidneys
3. _____ Accumulates as a result of anaerobic metabolism
4. _____ A potent vasodilator when produced in large quantities

II. Define the following terms.

Aerobic metabolism
Anaerobic metabolism
Anaphalactic shock
ARDS
Autotransfusion
Cardiac output
Cardiogenic shock
Central venous pressure
Disseminated intravascular clotting (DIC)
Hypovolemic shock
Intraarterial monitoring
Irreversible shock
MAST suit
Myocardial depressant factor
Neurogenic shock
Oliguria
Pulmonary artery pressure
Pulmonary capillary wedge pressure
Septic shock
Stroke volume
Vasoactive drugs
Vasogenic shock

III. Multiple choice

1. The underlying pathology in shock regardless of the type is:
  a. Anaerobic metabolism
  b. Decreased cardiac output
  c. Altered metabolism
  d. Tissue hypoperfusion

2. Which of the following factors is not associated with the etiology of shock?
   a. Alteration in the shape and size of the blood cells
   b. Inability of the heart to pump
   c. Excessive loss of intravascular fluids
   d. Interference with sympathetic impulses
3. The most common cause of hypovolemic shock is:
   a. Fluid loss from excessive vomiting and diarrhea
   b. Excessive blood loss
   c. Fluid shift to the third space
   d. Fluid loss from excessive diuresis
4. The most common cause of cardiogenic shock is:
   a. Myocardial infarction
   b. Cardiac tamponade
   c. Arrhythmias
   d. Pulmonary embolism
5. When shock occurs, which of the following findings would reflect the normal compensatory response of the heart?
   a. Oliguria
   b. Hypotension
   c. Bradycardia
   d. Tachycardia
6. When tachycardia occurs:
   a. The heart muscle needs less oxygen
   b. Oxygen supply to the heart muscle increases
   c. The diastolic period shortens
   d. Stroke volume remains unchanged
7. When vasogenic shock occurs:
   a. Blood pressure falls as a result of excessive loss of blood from intravascular spaces
   b. There is massive vasoconstriction as a result of increased sympathetic stimulation
   c. Cardiac output falls from the inability of the heart to pump blood.
   d. Venous return to the heart decreases as a result of loss of vasomotor tone
8. Which of the following is not a form of vasogenic shock?
   a. Septic shock
   b. Anaphylactic shock
   c. Neurogenic shock
   d. Hypovolemic shock
9. Excessive release of histamine causes:
   a. Vasodilation
   b. Vasoconstriction
10. The primary cause of septic shock is:
    a. Spinal anesthesia
    b. Pathogenic bacteria
    c. Exposure to an allergen
    d. Valvular disease
11. An early manifestation of septic shock that differentiates it from other types of shock would be:
    a. Decreased urinary output
    b. Decreased blood pressure
    c. Hypothermia
    d. Warm, flushed skin
12. During the early stages of shock, the compensatory responses that occur in the body as a result of sympathetic stimulation would be all *except*:
    a. Increased heart rate
    b. Dilation of blood vessels in the heart and brain
    c. Increased respiration
    d. Dilation of blood vessels to the skin, kidneys, and abdominal organs

13. Which of the following findings in a patient in shock would reflect the compensatory response to the renin-angiotensin system?
    a. Hyperkalemia
    b. Decreased urinary output
    c. Tachycardia
    d. Hypotension
14. Which of the following electrolyte imbalances occurs in shock as a result of metabolic acidosis?
    a. Intracellular hypokalemia
    b. Intravascular hypercalcemia
    c. Hypoproteinemia
    d. Hyponatremia
15. The primary effect resulting from lactic acid accumulation in the cells is:
    a. Fluid shift from interstitial to intravascular space
    b. Retention of nitrogenous products
    c. Fluid shift from intravascular to interstitial space
    d. Sodium and fluid retention in the intravascular space
16. Early manifestations of shock are:
    a. Altered level of consciousness and increased respirations
    b. Hypotension and tachycardia
    c. Restlessness and tachycardia
    d. Cool, clammy skin and hypotension
17. To obtain the most accurate assessment of fluid status of a patient in shock, the physician will look at:
    a. Blood pressure and pulse rate
    b. Patient's weight
    c. Central venous pressure readings
    d. Urinary output
18. A central venous pressure (CVP) reading reflects:
    a. Right atrial pressure
    b. Pulmonary capillary wedge pressure
    c. Pulmonary artery pressure
    d. Left atrial pressure
19. To obtain an accurate CVP reading, the nurse should:
    a. Position the patient so that the fluid in the manometer does not fluctuate with respirations
    b. Zero the manometer at the level of the patient's right atrium
    c. Change the patient's position when each reading is taken
    d. Place the manometer at the patient's left midaxillary line to take a reading
20. The nurse obtains a CVP reading of 10 cm of water. The nurse should:
    a. Notify the physician immediately
    b. Place the patient in a modified Trendelenburg position
    c. Check for accurate placement of CVP catheter
    d. Take no action
21. Fluid resuscitation for the patient in shock may be accomplished by all of the following interventions *except:*
    a. Use of the MAST suit
    b. Encouraging the patient to drink 2 to 3 L of fluid
    c. Administration of blood and blood products
    d. Use of various intravenous solutions
22. Which of the following drugs is not used in treating a patient in shock?
    a. Dobutamine
    b. Dopamine
    c. Allopurinol
    d. Nitroprusside

Charles Sullivan, age 52, is brought to the recovery room following major abdominal surgery. His estimated blood loss during surgery was 1200 ml. He received 1 unit of whole blood. His blood pressure is progressively falling, and his pulse rate is increasing. His abdominal dressing is saturated with a moderate amount of fresh sanguinous drainage. The nurse suspects the patient is developing shock and notifies the surgeon. Charles is semiconscious.

23. The physician orders an intravenous infusion of dopamine. In caring for Charles, the nurse should do all of the following *except:*
- **a.** Check his blood pressure every 5 to 15 minutes
- **b.** Use an infusion pump to administer the drug
- **c.** Observe the infusion site for signs of infiltration
- **d.** Discontinue the infusion immediately when Charles's blood pressure returns to normal limits

24. If the dopamine infusion should infiltrate, which of the following drugs would be most appropriate to use to counteract tissue necrosis?
- **a.** Regitine
- **b.** Naloxone
- **c.** Indomethacin
- **d.** Isoproterenol

25. Which of the following positions is appropriate for Charles?
- **a.** Sim's
- **b.** Semi-Fowler's
- **c.** Any position of comfort
- **d.** Flat with legs elevated

26. The nurse would suspect that Charles is recovering from shock when all of the following occur *except:*
- **a.** His pulse rate is between 60 and 100 beats/minute
- **b.** His urinary output is above 30 ml/hr
- **c.** His level of consciousness remains constant
- **d.** Mucous membranes are pink and skin is warm and dry

IV. Complete the following evaluation chart for a person who has been in shock.

Criteria to evaluate	Expected outcome
Activity	
Airway	
Respiratory status	
Cardiac status	
Communication	
CVP	
Blood gasses	
Freedom from infection	
Mucous membrane	
Rest	
Tissue Perfusion	
Freedom from injury	

Chapter 10

Pain

BRENDA GOODNER
VIVIENNE I. WALTON

CHAPTER OBJECTIVES

On completion of this chapter, the student should be able to:

- Describe the physiology of pain and the gate control theory of pain transmission.
- Compare factors that influence perception and reaction to pain.
- Identify analgesics effective for mild to moderate and moderate to severe pain, and factors to consider when giving narcotics.
- Describe medical approaches for pain control in addition to medications.
- Describe specific psychologic approaches for pain control.
- Identify guidelines for nursing interventions for pain control.
- Describe nursing measures to modify the pain stimulus and pain response.
- Explain the purpose and methods of the team approach for chronic pain control.

PREREQUISITE READING

Long-Phipps, Chapter 10, pp. 167-187.

Study thoroughly

1. Comparisons of acute and chronic pain
2. Comparisons of somatic and visceral pain

SELF-ASSESSMENT ACTIVITIES

I. Define the following terms.

Acetaminophen
Acetylsalicylic acid
Acupuncture
Acute pain
A-delta fibers
Ascending spinal pathways
B&O
Biofeedback
Brompton's solution
Causalgia
C fibers
Chronic pain
Cordotomy
Descending spinal pathways
Distraction
Endorphins
Gate control theory
Hyperalgesia
Hypnosis
Hypophysectomy
Intractable benign pain
Narcotic analgesics
Nerve block
Neuralgia
Neurectomy
Neuroaugmentation
Neurologic pain
Nociceptor
Nonnarcotic analgesics
Nonsteroidal antiinflammatory drugs
NSAIDS
OTC
PCA
PISCES
PQRST
Pain perception
Pain threshold
Pain tolerance
Phantom pain
Psychogenic pain
Referred pain
Rhizotomy
SG
SRT
STT
Serotinin
Substantia gelatinosa
Sympathectomy
TENS
Therapeutic touch
Visceral pain

II. Write your answers in the space provided.

1. How is pain transmitted?

2. How do endorphins suppress pain?

3. Briefly discuss the Gate Control Theory of pain transmission.

4. Pain threshold refers to ____________________.

5. Pain tolerance refers to ____________________.

6. What are factors that decrease pain tolerance?

7. What are factors that influence a person's reaction to pain?

8. What are the physiologic signs of pain?

9. Differentiate between chronic and acute pain.

10. In assessing pain, what does the mnemonic PQRST stand for?
    P:
    Q:
    R:
    S:
    T:

III. Multiple choice

1. Which of the following statements about pain is incorrect?
   a. Pain is a learned experience.
   b. Pain perception is the same among all persons.
   c. Pain is entirely a subjective phenomenon.
   d. The reaction to pain differs with each person.
2. A postsurgical patient states that she waits as long as she can before asking for her pain medication. The patient is describing her:
   a. Pain threshhold
   b. Pain perception
   c. Pain tolerance
   d. Addiction

3. Pain tolerance can be raised by all *except*:
   a. Application of heat or cold
   b. Gently rubbing the affected area
   c. Providing a quiet environment with little or no sensory input
   d. Providing distracting activities
4. In the gate control pain theory, the "gate" that "opens" and "closes" to control transmission of pain impulses is located in the:
   a. Substantia gelantinosa
   b. Thalamus
   c. Cortex
   d. Reticular-activating system
5. Which pain fibers conduct pain impulses at a rapid rate?
   a. C fibers
   b. A fibers
6. Pain perception occurs:
   a. At the site of the stimulus
   b. In the cerebral cortex
   c. From the preconceived ideas about illness
   d. From previous encounters with painful situations
7. A female patient states that she has gnawing, burning pain in her stomach after eating fried foods. The type of pain described by this patient is:
   a. Somatic
   b. Psychogenic
   c. Referred
   d. Visceral

Mr. Lambert, age 28, has had abdominal surgery. Today is his first postoperative day.

8. Mr. Lambert is requesting medication for pain. Which of the following assessments would be *least* important for the nurse to make prior to administering the medication for pain?
   a. Location of pain
   b. Intensity of pain
   c. Character of pain
   d. Cultural practices for pain
9. The nurse asks Mr. Lambert if his pain is sharp, dull, or burning. She is assessing:
   a. Reaction to pain
   b. Intensity of pain
   c. Character of pain
   d. Threshold of pain
10. The TENS unit and the spinal cord stimulator achieve pain control by:
    a. Altering electrical polarization of the electrolytes
    b. Stimulating the production of prostaglandins
    c. Blocking the transmission of the pain impulse
    d. Lowering the endorphin level
11. When a patient has a rhizotomy or cordotomy, the patient can expect pain relief:
    a. At the level of the incision
    b. Above the level of the incision
    c. All over the body
    d. Below the level of the incision
12. Which of the following are considered psychologic approaches for pain control?
    a. Behavior modification
    b. Biofeedback and autogenic training
    c. Hypnosis
    d. All of the above

13. Which of the following is incorrect as modifying the pain stimulus?
    a. Cutaneous stimulation; reduction of noise and visual stimuli
    b. Reduction of social isolation; therapeutic touch
    c. Distraction and relaxation exercises
    d. Pain therapies
14. Which of the following is considered as modifying the pain response?
    a. Explanation of the problem and decreasing anxiety
    b. Decreasing anxiety with medication
    c. Discouraging focus on the pain being experienced
    d. Detailed explanation about cultural patterns
15. The key to nursing implementation for a patient in pain is:
    a. Age and sex
    b. Cultural implications
    c. Source of the pain
    d. Individualized assessment
16. Pain is a subjective assessment. For the nurse treating the person in pain, this means:
    a. Pain depends on the physical source
    b. Pain must be physical to justify medications
    c. Objective data are essential in assessing pain
    d. Pain is whatever the patient says that it is
17. One of the most commonly used analgesic drugs is aspirin. The nurse must instruct the patient to take aspirin:
    a. Only on an empty stomach
    b. After meals or with a snack
    c. Two hours before meals
    d. Only between meals
18. The most common side effects of narcotics that the nurse must be alert for are:
    a. Increased respirations and blood pressure
    b. Increased respirations, bradycardia
    c. General depression of vital functions
    d. Hypotension, bradycardia, dyspnea
19. The nurse administering pain medications is aware that narcotics can be addicting. The nurse knows that research shows:
    a. Patients are easily addicted to narcotics
    b. Patients should not be given narcotics after 3 days
    c. Only terminal patients should get narcotic medications
    d. Less than 1% of patients become addicted in the hospital
20. Patient-controlled analgesia (PCA) is a method by which the patient can administer his own pain medication via a syringe pump. Studies show patients using PCA:
    a. Take twice as much pain medication
    b. Take less medication when not in pain
    c. Take pain medication when not in pain
    d. Take pain medication too frequently
21. The point at which the intensity of a stimulus causes a person to perceive pain is called:
    a. Pain tolerance
    b. Pain threshold
    c. Pain reception
    d. Acute pain
22. The nurse should recognize that the most widely accepted theory of pain transmission is the:
    a. Pattern theory
    b. Gate control theory
    c. Specificity theory
    d. Intensive theory

Tim Cabot, age 19, suffered a traumatic amputation of his left foot in a motorcycle accident. He is receiving meperidine (Demerol) 75 mg IM and acetaminophen (Tylenol) gr 10 PO every 3 hours for pain.

23. Tim complains of a burning sensation in his left foot. The nurse should explain that:
- **a.** This is a phantom pain that is not clearly understood
- **b.** This is not possible because his foot was amputated
- **c.** His regular pain medication will relieve the pain
- **d.** This phantom pain will disappear in about 1 week

24. One afternoon when Tim appears uncomfortable, the nurse asks if he wants his pain medication. Tim replies, "No, I'll wait until it gets really bad." The nurse's best response would be:
- **a.** "Okay. Ring when you're ready and I'll bring it right away."
- **b.** "If you let the pain get too severe, the medication will not work as well."
- **c.** "I admire you for your fortitude in facing pain."
- **d.** "Good, I'm glad you're concerned about too much medication."

Mr. John Andrew, 38, is admitted for evaluation and treatment of severe lower back pain. Mr. Andrew's admission orders include:

Regular diet
Out of bed as desired
Aspirin gr 10 PO every 3 hours prn for moderate pain
Aspirin gr 10 with codeine gr ½ PO every 3 hours for severe pain

Mr. Andrew received codeine and aspirin an hour ago and complains that he has experienced no relief.

25. The nurse's best initial action would be to:
- **a.** Explain that he cannot have more medication for 2 hours
- **b.** Call the physician for permission to repeat the medication
- **c.** Ask Mr. Andrew what measures other than drugs have helped relieve his pain
- **d.** Tell Mr. Andrew to be patient because the peak action of the medication is 90 minutes

26. Demerol is commonly used preoperatively. It is classified as a:
- **a.** Hypnotic
- **b.** Narcotic
- **c.** Drying agent
- **d.** Barbiturate

IV. Complete the following chart on each neurosurgical procedure for chronic intractable pain. The first has been done for you.

	Neurectomy	Rhizotomy	Cordotomy
Description of procedure	Resection of cranial or peripheral nerves supplying the affected area		
Clinical uses	Trigeminal neuralgia Incapacitating dysmenorrhea		
Contraindications	Not recommended for control of pain in the lower extremities because fibers that control movement and position sense are also resected during this procedure		
Residual effects	Peripheral nerve regeneration often requires repeat of the procedure		

V. Complete the following chart on nonnarcotic analgesics.

	Action	Adverse effects	Nursing considerations
Acetaminophen			
Ibuprofen			
Acetylsalicylic acid (aspirin)			
Propoxyphene (Darvon)			

VI. Complete the following chart on narcotic analgesics.

	Action	Adverse effects	Nursing considerations
Meperidine Hcl (Demerol)			
Morphine sulfate			
Codeine sulfate			
Hydromorphone (Dilaudid)			

VII. Write answer to the following directives in the space provided.

1. List the four pain theories. Briefly describe each theory.

2. List factors that influence an individual's reaction to pain.

VIII. Briefly discuss the following concepts.

1. Discuss why the following myths about pain relief are incorrect:
    1. Pain caused by anxiety doesn't require treatment.
    2. I've worked with enough patients to know which ones are really in pain.
    3. One way to determine whether a patient is faking is to give him a placebo.
    4. When a patient asks for pain medication every 4 hours on the dot, I know I've got a potential addict on my hands.
    5. The patient who needs an increasing dose of narcotics to control pain is becoming an addict.
    6. Giving analgesics only on demand is the best way to prevent abuse.
    7. The best injectable narcotic for pain relief is meperidine.
2. Discuss the seven major guidelines for pain relief measures.
    1. Preparation for painful experiences
    2. Preventive approach
    3. Placebo response
    4. Patient's ability or will to participate
    5. Varying pain relief measures
    6. Introducing new pain relief measures
    7. Giving analgesics
3. For your consideration:
    1. How do you view pain?
    2. Have you been assigned to a patient experiencing pain? What were your thoughts and feelings toward the patient during the pain experience?

DIRECTIONS FOR RESEARCH

Are nurses using independent measures such as repositioning, gentle rubbing of the affected area, or distraction in conjunction with the administration of pain medication or are they just administering the pain medication? Data for this type of study can best be obtained through direct observation. Select clinical units that routinely care for patients with problems that are normally associated with pain, such as a surgical unit, an orthopedic unit, or an oncology unit. When patients on the unit are given pain medication, accompany the nurse administering the medication to the patient's room to observe if any independent pain relief measures were used.

CLINICAL ACTIVITY

Is there a pain clinic in your community? If so, plan a visit to find out what interventions are being used in pain management. What is the role of the nurse in the pain clinic?

SUGGESTED READINGS

Barnhouse, AH and others: Evaluation of acute pain: a comparison of patient and nurse perspectives (research), J Nurs Qual Assur 2(3):54-63, 1988.

Bast, C, and Hayes, P: PCA: a new way to spell pain relief, RN 49:18-20, Aug 1986.

Pain-controlled analgesia allows patient to administer his own postoperative pain medication and thereby maintain a constant blood level and more effective pain relief. The author explains what to teach the patient, safety features of the unit to prevent abuse, and potential applications for PCA for use with any chronic pain condition.

Blake, CJ: Morphine: new route for better pain relief, Nursing 18(3):111, 1988.

Bondestam, E, and others: Pain assessment by patients and nurses in the early phase of acute myocardial infarction, J Adv Nurs 12(6):677-682, 1987.

Brucker, MC: Management of common minor discomfort in pregnancy: managing minor pain in pregnancy (Part II), J Nurse Midwife, 33(1):25-30, 1988.

Domask, ME, and others: Patient and nurse perceptions of analgesic and administration times (research), J Qual Assur 2(3):64-69, 1988.

Escobar, PL: Management of chronic pain, Nurse Pract 10:24-32, Jan 1985.

Describes the pathophysiology of pain, diagnostic tests, and therapeutic interventions (drugs, relaxation, biofeedback, hypnosis, acupuncture, transcutaneous nerve stimulator, nerve blocks, trigger point blocks, heat/cold applications, behavior modification, surgical procedures, placebos, and pain clinics).

Kahn, AB: Narcotic analgesics and antagonist. In Mosby's Pharmacology in nursing, St Louis, 1986, The CV Mosby Co.

Kahn, AB: Nonsteroidal antiinflammatory agents and nonnarcotic analgesics. In Mosby's pharmacology in nursing, St Louis, 1986, The CV Mosby Co.

Kleinke, CL, and others: Predicting treatment outcomes of chronic back pain patients in a multidisciplinary pain clinic: methodological issues and treatment implications, Pain 33(1):41-48, 1988.

Lierman, LM: Phantom breast experiences after mastectomy (research), Onocol Nurs Forum 15(1):41-44, 1988.

McCaffery, M, and Beebe, A: Pain: clinical manual for nursing practice, St Louis, 1989, The CV Mosby Co.

McGuire, L: Seven myths about pain relief, RN, 46:30-31, Dec. 1983.

Rodgers, J: Pains of complaint: do patients' cries for relief actually make them feel worse? Psychol Today, 22(4):26-27, 1988.

Rose, V: The misery of pain, Geriatr Nurs Home Care 7(12):24-25, 1987.

Wallace, L: Psychological aspects of physical illness: chronic pelvic pain, Nurs Time 83(50):45-47, 1987.

Chapter 11

Infection Control

CAROLE KAUFMANN

CHAPTER OBJECTIVES

On completion of this chapter, the student should be able to:

- Describe the chain of infection.
- Identify high-risk factors for infection.
- Describe white blood cell response to infection.
- Identify community approaches to infection control and describe immunization programs.
- Define nosocomial infections and measures of prevention and control (bacteremia, urinary, wound, and respiratory infections).
- Identify two systems of isolation precautions and describe general approaches for each.

PREREQUISITE READING

Long-Phipps, Chapter 11, pp. 189-211.

SELF-ASSESSMENT ACTIVITIES

I. Define the following terms.

Active immunization
AHA
AIDS
Booster dose
Carriers
CDC
Communicable disease
DPT
Herd immunity
Incubation period
Infection
Inoculation
Invasiveness
JCAH
MMR
Nosocomial infection
Passive immunization
Pathogen
Pathogenicity
Protective isolation
TOPV
Toxigenicity

II. Identify these key terms.

Abscess
Acquired immunity
Antibody
Antigen
Attenuated live vaccine
B cell
Bacteremia
Cell-mediated immune response
Cellulitis
Chemotaxis
Complement
Gamma globulin
Humoral immune response
Immunity
Immunization
Immunoglobulins
Inflammatory response
Interferon
Killed vaccine
Leukocytosis
Lymphadenitis
Lymph node
Lymphocyte
Lysozyme
Macrophage
Natural immunity
Phagocytosis
Scar tissue
Sedimentation rate
Self versus nonself
Septicemia
T cell
Toxoid
Vaccine

III. Multiple choice

1. The first doctor to advocate and demonstrate the significance of handwashing to combat the transmission of infection was:

a. Felming
b. Semmelweiss
c. Lister
d. Koch

2. Hospital-acquired infections are called:

a. Penicillin-resistant infections
b. Secondary infections
c. Nosocomial infections
d. Transplacental infections

3. The chain of infection involves:

a. Causative agent, reservoir, portal of exit, mode of transmission, portal of entry, and susceptible host
b. Helminth, incubation period, symptomatic clinical symptoms, colonization, and superinfection
c. Age, reservoir, blood, mode of transmission, colonization, and superinfection
d. Susceptible host, mode of transmission, portal of exit, incubation period, colonization, and mode of entry

4. Examples of modes of transmission of infection are:

a. Age, impaired immune status, contact and airborne
b. Poor nutritional status, age, vehicle and vector
c. Impaired skin integrity, airborne, vector, contact
d. Contact, airborne, vehicle and vector

5. In assessing a patient, a nurse would be alert to suspect an infection when:

a. WBC count is 5000 to 10,000 WBC/mm^3
b. WBC count is 10,000 to 20,000 WBC/mm^3
c. RBC count is 5000 to 10,000 RBC/mm^3
d. RBC count is 10,000 to 20,000 RBC/mm^3

6. To confirm a diagnosis of infection, the nurse is asked to take a culture of the infected site. The best time to take the culture is:

a. 8 AM as soon as laboratory opens
b. Before starting antibiotics
c. After starting antibiotics
d. Any time, because cultures are unaffected by antibiotics

7. Whether a pathogenic organism causes an infection once it enters the body is primarily dependent upon all *except:*

a. Host susceptibility
b. Dose of the agent
c. Mode of transmission
d. Duration and intimacy of contact

8. Infection prevention and control measures in the community would include all *except:*

a. Immunizations
b. Water and sewage sanitation programs
c. Monitoring handwashing practices of children in schools
d. Monitoring sanitation practices of food handlers

Mr. Zeiken underwent abdominal surgery 3 days ago. His abdominal dressing is to be changed prn.

9. The nurse should suspect that Mr. Zeiken is developing an infection in his surgical wound when she detects all of the following *except:*

a. Purulent drainage from the incision
b. Persistent redness and swelling of the incision
c. The formation of granulation tissue at the incision
d. Increased incisional pain

10. The nurse would suspect that Mr. Zeiken is developing a generalized infection when he experienced all *except:*
    a. Fever
    b. Elevated WBC
    c. Malaise
    d. Diaphoresis
11. Which diagnostic test would provide the most accurate information about the organism causing Mr. Zeiken's wound infection?
    a. Urinalysis
    b. Gastric analysis
    c. Blood culture
    d. Wound culture
12. Which of the following agencies is responsible for programs for the prevention and control of communicable diseases and other preventable diseases in the United States?
    a. WHO
    b. CDC
    c. JCAH
    d. AHA
13. Immunization programs are important in controlling infectious diseases throughout the world. You have been asked to explain the effects of DPT to a new mother. Your best response would be:
    a. "It will stimulate your baby's body to produce its own antibodies, and the baby will need booster shots."
    b. "It will give your baby all the antibodies it will need, but the baby will need a booster."
    c. "It will give your baby all the antibodies it will need, and the baby will need no booster."
    d. "It is not really necessary, since the United States does not have smallpox."
14. The nurse is responsible for assessing persons before immunizations because:
    a. Some people do not like to take medications by mouth
    b. Some people are allergic to milk
    c. Some people are allergic to dogs and cats
    d. Some people are allergic to eggs
15. The most common nosocomial infection seen in the hospital is:
    a. Common cold
    b. Clostridium
    c. Urinary tract infection
    d. Deep wound infection
16. In obtaining a sterile urine specimen from a client with an indwelling catheter attached to a closed drainage system, the method of choice for collecting the specimen is:
    a. With sterile gloves, disconnect the catheter from the tubing, take the specimen, then carefully reconnect the catheter and tubing.
    b. Obtain the specimen with a sterile needle and syringe through the rubber portal, using aseptic technique.
    c. Using aseptic technique, wash the urinary meatus, then push the catheter into the bladder as far as it will go to collect a new specimen.
    d. Clamp off the catheter, disconnect the catheter at the proximal drainage tube junction, and collect the specimen under sterile conditions.
17. Indwelling catheters should be changed:
    a. Every 3 days
    b. Every 5 days
    c. Once a week
    d. Only when they become obstructed
18. The nosocomial infection that is associated with the highest mortality is:
    a. Pneumonia
    b. Surgical infection
    c. Urinary tract infection
    d. Gastroenteritis

19. Strict isolation means:
- **a.** Door is closed
- **b.** Mask is worn by everyone
- **c.** Gloves are worn by everyone
- **d.** All of the above

20. Intravenous and intraarterial catheters should be changed:
- **a.** Every 24 hours
- **b.** Every 24 to 36 hours
- **c.** Every 48 to 72 hours
- **d.** Every 80 to 86 hours

21. Used needles should be discarded by:
- **a.** Placing them (after recapping) in designated puncture-resistant containers
- **b.** Placing uncapped in designated puncture-resistant containers
- **c.** Bending, so they cannot be used again
- **d.** Detaching them from the syringes, then discarding in designated puncture-resistant containers

22. Enteric precautions are designated to prevent infections that are transmitted by contact with:
- **a.** Feces
- **b.** Blood
- **c.** Urine
- **d.** Purulent drainage from wound

23. Masks should be worn:
- **a.** Over nose and mouth, used only once
- **b.** Over mouth only, used only once
- **c.** Over nose and mouth, then stored around neck
- **d.** Over mouth only, then stored around neck

24. The most important measure in preventing cross-infections is:
- **a.** Using rubber gloves
- **b.** Using gown and gloves
- **c.** Using masks
- **d.** Handwashing

25. Your patient has been placed on BSI (body specimen isolation). This means that:
- **a.** Gloves are to be used only when giving intramuscular injections.
- **b.** Linen is to be disposed of by the usual method.
- **c.** Gloves are to be used when handling all specimens.
- **d.** All used needles must be recapped before discarding.

SUGGESTED READINGS

AIDS precautions and changing practice, RNs agree; OSHA already moving to enforce CDC guidelines, Am J Nurs 88(3):373, 388, 390, 1988.

Pritchard, V: Geriatric infections: the gastrointestinal tract, RN 1988 Apr., 51(4):58-60.

Preventing infections transmitted by contact, Nursing 18(3):112, 1988.

Recommendations for preventing transmission of HIV in health care settings, Can Med Assoc J 138(3):213-219, 1988.

Chapter 12
Cancer

MARY S. NICHOLS

CHAPTER OBJECTIVES

On completion of this chapter, the student should be able to:

- Discuss the epidemiologic variables related to cancer and the nurse's role in cancer epidemiology.
- Outline the pathophysiology of malignant tumors, focusing on the concepts of tumor growth and metastasis.
- List several factors that contribute to carcinogenesis.
- Describe the nurse's role in cancer prevention and health education.
- Conduct a holistic assessment of the oncology patient and identify appropriate nursing diagnoses.
- Explain the rationale for four categories of cancer therapy and discuss nursing interventions for patients receiving those therapies.
- Formulate a plan of care for the patient with advanced cancer.

PREREQUISITE READING

Long-Phipps, Chapter 12, pp. 213-261.

SELF-ASSESSMENT ACTIVITIES

I. Define the following terms.

Anaplasia
Cachexia
Cell cycle time
Cell differentiation
Dysplasia
Flare reaction
Hyperplasia
Hypertrophy
Metaplasia
Mitosis
Oncogenes
Pallative treatment
Stomatitis

II. Complete the chart below. For each of the sites listed, write the early warning signals of cancer.

Site	Early warning signals
Breast	
Colon	
Lung	
Oral cavity	
Skin	
Uterus	
Kidney and bladder	
Larynx	
Prostate gland	
Stomach	

III. Multiple choice

1. The leading cause of cancer death in women involves the:
   - **a.** Lungs
   - **b.** Ovaries
   - **c.** Uterus
   - **d.** Breast
2. The leading cause of cancer death in men involves the:
   - **a.** Lungs
   - **b.** Penis
   - **c.** Prostate gland
   - **d.** Kidney
3. The leading cause of cancer death in children and adolescents is:
   - **a.** Cancer of the brain
   - **b.** Hodgkin's disease
   - **c.** Leukemia
   - **d.** Cancer of the bone

4. The role of the nurse in cancer prevention includes all *except:*
   a. Case finding
   b. Health teaching
   c. Genetic counseling
   d. Prescribing treatments
5. Which of the following factors is least likely to interfere with cancer health-seeking behavior?
   a. Lack of education
   b. A positive attitude toward the disease
   c. Fear of social disgrace
   d. Reliance on unproven, quick, painless cure methods
6. Normal cell mitosis occurs in which of the following sequences?
   a. Telophase, metaphase, prophase, anaphase
   b. Prophase, metaphase, anaphase, telophase
   c. Metaphase, telophase, prophase, anaphase
   d. Anaphase, prophase, telophase, metaphase
7. Benign tumors differ from malignant tumors in that malignant tumors:
   a. Do not invade surrounding tissue
   b. Do not recur once surgically removed
   c. Proliferate rapidly
   d. Involve proliferation of mature cells
8. The type of malignant cells that have the worse prognosis and the highest degree of malignancy are those that:
   a. Are very similar to the tissue of origin
   b. Are some what similar to the tissue of origin
   c. Have little similarity to the tissue of origin
   d. Grow very slowly in a limited area
9. Factors affecting the growth of neoplasms include all *except:*
   a. The existence of an immune surveillance system
   b. Whether the tumor tissue is regulated by sex hormones
   c. Whether stem cells evolve
   d. The age of the host
10. Characteristic findings of malignant cells include all *except:*
    a. Loss of differentiation
    b. Large, irregularly shaped nuclei
    c. Proliferation throughout the body
    d. Encapsulation
11. Which class of tumor has the worse prognosis?
    a. Grade 1
    b. Grade 2
    c. Grade 3
    d. Grade 4
12. Metastasis of a tumor occurs through all of the following ways *except:*
    a. Blood stream
    b. Sexual intercourse
    c. Lymphatic system
    d. Direct extension
13. All of the following methods have been used to classify tumors *except:*
    a. Cell type origin
    b. Cell maturity
    c. Scientist who first discovered them
    d. Survival rate
14. Preventive measures against cancer include all *except:*
    a. Teaching people to reduce dietary intake of fiber
    b. Teaching people to adhere to safety practices in the work environment
    c. Encouraging people to stop smoking
    d. Encouraging regular physical examinations

15. The only definitive way that cancer can be diagnosed is by:
    a. Ultrasound
    b. Biopsy
    c. CT scan
    d. Measuring serum enzymes
16. When planning care for the patient with cancer, which of the following questions would be more important?
    a. How is the patient's appetite?
    b. Does the patient have problems with elimination?
    c. Does the patient know the diagnosis?
    d. What is the patient's level of physical activity?
17. When caring for a patient who has internal radiotherapy, the caregiver can be protected from overexposure to radiation by observing the principles of all of the following *except:*
    a. Time
    b. Site
    c. Distance
    d. Shielding
18. A patient on chemotherapy will require dosage adjustment when which of the following occurs?
    a. Alopecia
    b. Nausea and vomiting
    c. Bone marrow suppression
    d. Stomatitis

IV. Write your answers in the space provided.

1. Why is the survival rate for cancer much higher today than it was years ago?

2. What are the three leading sites of cancer?

3. List the seven warning signals of cancer.

4. What has been the focus of cancer nursing research?

5. What are the functions of the American Cancer Society?

6. List some cancer patient groups. What is the primary function of any cancer patient group?

7. What does the abbreviation TNM stand for? How is the TNM classification system used in cancer care?

8. Write down one type of cancer that is purely hereditary.

9. To provide a shield against exposure to radiation, of what must the material worn by the caregiver be made?

10. Why must patients have several or more courses of chemotherapy?

11. What is Brompton's cocktail? What is it used for?

V. Complete the chart below on chemotherapy agents. List the major classifications, indicate by (✓) if the class is cell cycle specific or nonspecific, state the mode of action, and give a minimum of two examples of each.

Classification	Cell cycle		Mode of action	Examples
	Specific	Nonspecific		

VI. Select the best answer for each item.

1. Interferon's antitumor effect is based on its ability to:
   a. Strengthen the body's natural killer (NK) cells
   b. Prevent the synthesis of DNA in tumor cells
   c. Directly inhibit cell replication
   d. Block absorption of nutrients by tumor cells

Mrs. Langhorn has advanced ovarian cancer. She is scheduled for cobalt treatments to the pelvic area.

2. Which side effect is Mrs. Langhorn least likely to experience from radiotherapy?
   a. Diarrhea
   b. Cystitis
   c. Pneumonitis
   d. Fatigue

3. When assisting Mrs. Langhorn with hygienic care, you observe a red square marking over the suprapubic area. You should:
   a. Avoid washing off the marking
   b. Apply a thin film of vaseline inside the square before she goes for her cobalt treatment
   c. Ask the x-ray technicians to remove the marking, since they put it on
   d. Understand that the area within the square will not be exposed to radiation
4. Five days after cobalt treatment, Mrs. Langhorn's suprapubic skin surface is red and very tender to touch. You should:
   a. Avoid washing the affected area until you receive instructions from the radiologist
   b. Apply A & D ointment to the affected area
   c. Understand that this finding indicates that the cancer has metastasized to the skin
   d. Apply an antibiotic ointment because an infection is present
5. Phase-specific chemotherapy drugs are most effective with tumor cells that:
   a. Divide rapidly
   b. Divide slowly
6. To maintain patency of a Hickman catheter, you should:
   a. Change the caps daily
   b. Irrigate the catheter with a solution of heparinized saline
   c. Avoid taping the catheter to the patient's chest
   d. Aspirate and discard a small quantity of blood daily
7. The primary reason that side effects of chemotherapy classically involve the bone marrow, the GI tract, and the hair follicles is that each of these types of tissue is:
   a. Composed of aged cells
   b. Composed of immature cells
   c. Composed of cells that divide slowly
   d. Composed of cells that divide rapidly
8. An individual on chemotherapy has a neutrophil count of $1000/mm^3$. Which nursing diagnosis would be most appropriate?
   a. Potential for injury
   b. Potential for fluid volume deficit
   c. Potential for alterations in nutrition
   d. Potential for infection
9. Which statement about immunotherapy is incorrect?
   a. It is most effective as a primary treatment of large inoperable tumors.
   b. Its use is limited to the control of selective types of small tumors.
   c. It is based on a premise that cancer cells are perceived by the body as antigens.
   d. It is dependent upon the body producing T cells and B cells.
10. Medication to control pain in patients with advanced cancer would:
    a. Be given prn starting with the highest dose prescribed
    b. Always be given IM or IV
    c. Be tightly controlled to prevent addiction
    d. Be administered on a regularly scheduled basis
11. Which statement about hospice is incorrect?
    a. It is a place where cancer patients can go to die.
    b. It is a program of care designed to meet the needs of the dying patient and family.
    c. Its primary emphasis is on home care.
    d. It involves care 24 hours a day, 7 days a week.
12. Psychologic support of the patient with advanced cancer would involve:
    a. Helping the patient develop a sense of detachment from the family in preparation for death
    b. Helping the patient accept that his or her situation is hopeless
    c. Helping the patient find a reason for living
    d. Helping the patient understand why he or she is being punished

13. Cancer cachexia is:
    a. Characterized by progressive wasting
    b. A form of starvation
    c. A form of protein-calorie malnutrition
    d. An early manifestation of cancer
14. Which type of rays has the greatest depth of penetration?
    a. Alpha
    b. Gamma
    c. Beta
    d. Delta
15. Which of the following is not a method of immunotherapy?
    a. Administration of BCG vaccine
    b. Transferring lymphocytes from one tumor patient to another
    c. Administration of tetrahydrocannabinol (THC)
    d. Administration of interferon

VII. Write your response to the questions that follow each situation.

1. A patient with cancer of the thyroid gland is given radioactive iodine orally.
    a. Will isolation be required? Why or why not?

    b. What are the sources of contamination?

    c. What would you do if the patient vomits and soils the bed linen?

2. A patient with advanced cancer of the lung is given radioactive gold, which has been injected directly into the pleural cavity. A day later the patient dies.
    a. What are the sources of contamination?

    b. How would you know that there has been leakage of radioactive material from the pleural cavity?

    c. If there is leakage, what should you do?

    d. What precautions must you take before the body is transported to the morgue?

3. A female patient with cancer of the uterus has radium implanted into the uterus. She is on bedrest until the implant is removed in 2 days. She also has a Foley catheter in place.
   a. What are the sources of contamination?

   b. What precautions should you take in caring for her?

VIII. Briefly discuss the following concepts.

1. Diseases that are characterized by production of abnormal cells that do not obey the laws of tissue growth
2. Why one out of every two persons with cancer can survive
3. How malignant cells differ from normal cells
4. How cancer spreads on the body
5. An individual's risk of developing cancer at age 60
6. The factors that contribute to carcinogens
7. The most common sites of cancer in women and men
8. The broad range of psychotic responses
9. Treatment modalities such as surgery, radiotherapy, chemotherapeutic drugs, and biologic response modifiers
10. The four reasons for higher prevalence of cancer among black people

IX. Reminder to student: answer all the items in the "Putting knowledge to practice" box on p. 165 of text.

CASE STUDY

Mr. Gerard Allison, 52 years of age, has metastatic cancer of the prostate gland. He is receiving chemotherapy and has experienced all of the following problems listed in the care plan below. Complete the care plan for him.

	Nursing diagnosis	**Goals**	**Interventions (include preventive and corrective)**
Dryness of mouth and stomatitis			
Anorexia and weight loss			
Nausea and vomiting			
Diarrhea			
Constipation			

Continued

	Nursing diagnosis	Goals	Interventions (include preventive and corrective)
Alopecia			
Fatigue and anemia			
Leukopenia			
Thrombocytopenia			
Neurotoxicity			
Pain			
Cystitis			
Extravasation of a vesicant			
Extravasation of a nonvesicant			

CLINICAL ACTIVITIES

1. Is there a cancer registry in your community? If so, plan a visit to find out what their methods of cancer surveillance are and what their role is in the management of cancer.
2. Plan a visit to the American Cancer Society to find out what services they provide for cancer patients.
3. What cancer patient groups are available in your community?
4. What are your thoughts and feelings about caring for patients with metastatic cancer?
5. Choose a group, decide on a format, and share insights from nursing literature and the mass media on perspectives in cancer. This could be a beginning "Nurse's Journal Club."
6. Role-play a nursing interview assessment for a person diagnosed as having cancer (of the cervix, breast, lungs, prostate rectum, and so on). Expand the various roles of health team and family.
7. What are the innovations that you would activate for yourself, family, and community (or group) in relation to cancer prevention?
8. Formulate specific assessment questions related to diagnosis of cancer, using a recent guide assessment. For example, the first step is to determine whether the patient knows the diagnosis of cancer. Next, assess what the patient has been told by the doctor, health team or family. (See p. 232 of text.)

SUGGESTED READINGS

Barston, J: Hormonal therapy for patients with advanced cancer, Home Health Nurse 4:43-45, March-April, 1986.
Describes type of patients who might benefit from hormonal therapy, side effects of therapy, and what to do.

Crosley, MA: Watch out for nutritional complications of cancer, RN 48:22-26, Mar 1985.
Describes how malnutrition and protein-calorie deficiencies develop in cancer. Provides a quick guide to detecting vitamin-mineral deficiencies, and a care plan that focuses on meeting the dietary needs of cancer patients.

Hahn, AB, and others: Drugs used in neoplastic disease. In Mosby's pharmacology in nursing, St. Louis, 1986, The CV Mosby Co.

Hickey, SS: Enabling hope, Cancer Nurs 9:133-137, June 1986.
Excellent article. Defines hope and enabling. Explains why people need hope and nursing approaches for enabling hope.

Lindsey, A: Cancer cachexia: effects of disease and its treatment, Seminars in Oncology Nursing 2:19-29, Feb 1986.
Describes incidence and prevalence of cachexia, manifestations and consequences, theories of pathogenesis, and the effects of cancer treatment on the development of cachexia.

Ostchega, Y, and Culane, M: Tumor markets: Key pieces to your cancer patient's clinical picture, Nursing 15:48-51, Sept 1985.
Defines tumor markers and their value in diagnosing, evaluating prognosis, and monitoring cancer patient's response to treatment. Provides a chart showing the common tumor markers and the significance of each.

Williams, SR: Nutrition and cancer. In Nutrition and dietary therapy, St. Louis, 1989, The CV Mosby Co.

Chapter 13
Substance Abuse

VIVIENNE I. WALTON

CHAPTER OBJECTIVES

On completion of this chapter, the student should be able to:

- Name four negative compulsions that are considered addictions.
- Define the difference between tolerance (behavioral, pharmacologic, and cross tolerance) and dependence (physical, psychologic, and cross dependence).
- Name one legal effort and one educational effort to prevent alcoholism and chemical dependency.
- Define the term *enabling* and term *intervention.*
- State two theories of the development of alcoholism.
- Name five disorders directly associated with alcoholism.
- Discuss alcohol withdrawal, including delirium tremens, and actions taken to prevent or reduce withdrawal.
- Define drug addiction and drug habituation.
- Name the six basic types of drugs, citing examples, how they are used, street names, effects and side effects, pathophysiology, and symptoms of overdose.
- Discuss why nurses are at increased risk for chemical dependency.

PREREQUISITE READING

Long-Phipps, Chapter 13, pp. 263-289.

SELF-ASSESSMENT ACTIVITIES

I. Define the following terms.

Anxiety attack
Behavior modification
Blackouts
Blood alcohol level
Chemical dependency
Cocaine crash
Craving
Deliriants
Delirium tremens
Delusions
Depressant
Detox
Detoxification
Drug addiction
Drug habituation
Empty calories
Enabling
Enabling behavior
Fetal alcohol syndrome
Flashbacks
Grand mal seizures
Hallucinations
Inhaling
Intervention
Impaired nurse
Mild tremors
Myopathies
Narcolepsy
Neuropathy
Physical dependency
Planned confrontations
Positive reinforcement
Problem drinkers
Psychologic dependency
Raising the bottom
Sedative hypnotics
Severe agitation
Substance abuse
Tolerance
Wernicke-Korsakoff's syndrome
Withdrawal

II. Match the etiologic theory of alcoholism with the appropriate description.

a. Oral fixation
b. Genetic theory
c. Genetotropic theory
d. Behavioral learning theory
e. Endocrine theory
f. Sociocultural theory

1. _____ Alcoholism is related to a genetically determined biochemical defect.
2. _____ The association of alcohol ingestion with a positive experience.
3. _____ Alcoholism is directly related to cultural attitudes and stress factors.
4. _____ Alcoholism is hereditary.
5. _____ Alcoholism is caused by a pituitary-adrenocortical deficiency that results in hypoglycemia.
6. _____ Alcoholism is caused by absence of warmth and nurturing during the oral stage of development.

III. Match the organization with the appropriate persons

a. AA (Alcoholics Anonymous)
b. Al-Anon
c. Al-Ateen

1. _____ Self-help organization for spouses of alcoholics
2. _____ Self-help organization for alcoholic youths
3. _____ Self-help organization for alcoholics

IV. Match the drugs listed below with the appropriate classification

a. Stimulants
b. Narcotics
c. Depressants
d. Cannabis
e. Hallucinogens
f. Deliriant

1. _____ amphetamines
2. _____ heroin
3. _____ marijuana
4. _____ mescaline
5. _____ tranquilizers
6. _____ aerosol sprays
7. _____ codeine
8. _____ nicotine
9. _____ PCP
10. _____ methadone
11. _____ sedatives
12. _____ caffeine
13. _____ anesthetics
14. _____ LSD
15. _____ meperidine
16. _____ hashish
17. _____ solvents
18. _____ morphine
19. _____ barbiturates

V. Multiple choice

1. Theories concerning the cause of alcoholism include:
  a. Psychologic theories
  b. Physiologic theories
  b. Cultural-etiologic and sociocultural theories
  d. All of the above

2. In substance abuse, dependency refers to:
   a. Physical dependency
   b. Psychologic dependency
   c. Psychologic and physical dependency
   d. Neurologic impairment
3. Medical disorders associated with alcoholism are:
   a. Neurologic and cardiovascular
   b. Musculoskeletal and immunologic
   c. Hepatic and gastrointestinal
   d. All of the above
4. The legal limit for intoxication, according to most laws, is a blood alcohol level of
   a. 100 mg/100 ml
   b. 50 mg/100 ml
   c. 75 mg/100 ml
   d. 25 mg/100 ml
5. Manifestations of alcohol withdrawal would include all except:
   a. Nausea or vomiting, hallucinations
   b. Restlessness, anorexia, convulsions
   c. Signs of vasomotor lability
   d. Diaphoresis, tachycardia, elevated blood pressure
6. Which of the following behaviors exhibited by a patient would *not* be considered as DTs?
   a. Pleasant, relaxed state, loosening of inhibitions
   b. Confusion and disorientation
   c. Fearfulness and tachycardia
   d. Temperature elevation (100° to 105°)
7. Manifestations of fetal alcohol syndrome include:
   a. Mental retardation
   b. Malformations of skeletal and urogenic systems
   c. Microcephaly and growth deficiencies
   d. All of the above
8. Routine diagnostic blood tests that often reveal abnormalities that are directly related to alcoholism include:
   a. SGOT and SGPT
   b. SGOT
   c. SGPT
   d. None of the above
9. Medications used in the initial period of detoxification include which of the following?
   a. Chlordiazepoxide (Librium)
   b. Phenytoin (Dilantin)
   c. Magnesium sulfate and multivitamins
   d. All of the above
10. Teaching for the patient with alcoholism includes which of the following?
    a. Drugs to avoid and products that contain alcohol
    b. Importance of aftercare, including AA
    c. Signs and symptoms of impending relapse
    d. All of the above
11. Which is the exception for manifestations of nicotine withdrawal symptoms?
    a. Constipation, diarrhea
    b. Headaches, fatigue, insomnia
    c. Sense of confidence and well-being
    d. Impairment of psychomotor performance

12. Amphetamines are considered CNS stimulants. Which is not considered a side-effect of amphetamine usage?
    - a. Suppression of appetite
    - b. Restlessness, dizziness
    - c. Insomnia, headache
    - d. Diarrhea, constipation
13. Which of the following would not be exhibited in cocaine psychosis?
    - a. Hallucinations, insomnia
    - b. Loss of pleasure
    - c. Breathing difficulty
    - d. Increased potential for violence
14. Which medication would be administered to a patient for methaqualone withdrawal?
    - a. Atropine sulfate or Dilantin
    - b. Antabuse or Narcan
    - c. Diazepam or phenobarbital
    - d. Benzedrine or methadone
15. Which are the common types of tranquilizers found in the benzodiazepine family?
    - a. Valium, Librium
    - b. Serax, Atarax
    - c. Ativan, Tranxene
    - d. All of the above
16. The most prominent toxic effect of delirants is:
    - a. Depression of the central nervous system
    - b. Euphoric sensations
    - c. Increased restlessness and excitability
    - d. Liver damage
17. Which statement about cannabis is correct?
    - a. The drug is associated with severe withdrawal reactions.
    - b. Patients experience acute "flashback" episodes after use of the drug is discontinued.
    - c. Overdose is treated with naloxone (Narcan).
    - d. Persons develop a psychologic dependency to the drug.

VI. Fill in the blanks:

a. Flashbacks	**e.** Clonidine
b. Crack	**f.** Stomach
c. Magnesium	**g.** Intestine
d. Depressant	**h.** Major and minor

1. Alcohol is a central nervous system _____ .
2. Alcohol is absorbed in both the _____ and _____ .
3. _____ is often decreased in persons who are alcoholic, usually because of poor dietary intake.
4. The National Council on Alcoholism divides alcoholism into _____ criteria systems.
5. _____ is more addicting than other forms of cocaine.
6. _____ may occur in the use of hallucinogens.
7. _____ is often used for the purpose of detoxification from narcotics.

CLINICAL ACTIVITIES

1. What is the legal limit of blood alcohol level for driving in your state?
2. What organizations or groups are available in your community to provide support for the alcoholic and the drug abuser? Plan a visit to these organizations or groups to find out what services they provide?
3. Visit a drug store and make a list of mouthwashes and liquid over-the-counter medications that contain alcohol.
4. Is there an impaired nurse program in your state? What does it consist of?

SUGGESTED READINGS

Adams, FE: Drug dependency in hospital patients, Am J Nurs 88(4):477-481, 1988.

Allen, JR, and others: Prevention of AIDS and HIV infection: needs and priorities for epidemiologic research, Am J Publ Health 78(4):381-386, 1988.

Baguali, G: Education on drugs and alcohol: past disappointments and future challenges, Health Educ Res 2(4):417-422, 1987.

Knot, DH, and others: Acute withdrawal from alcohol: diagnosis and treatment, Emerg Med 20(5):271-281, 1988.

Lachman, VD: The chemically dependent nurse, Holist Nurse Pract 2(4):34-44, 1988.

Lancelotta, PB: Inauguration of a chemical dependency rehabilitation unit: supplying the nursing component. Nurs Manage 19(1):32R-32T, 1988.

McNeely, E: Drug testing: ethical considerations, J Am Assoc Occup Health Nurs 36(3):118, 120, 1988.

Powell, AH: Alcohol withdrawal syndrome, Am J Nurs 88(3):312-315, 1988.

Roach, WH, Jr, and others: Confidentiality of alcohol and drug abuse patient records: the 1987 regulations, Am Med Rec Assoc 59(4):28-39, 1988.

Talashek, ML: Parental alcoholism and adolescent ego-identity, Community Health Nurs 4(4):211-212, 1987.

Wade, M: Meeting the challenge of alcohol and drug abuse in older adults, Home Health Care Nurs 5(5):19, 22-23, 1987.

Chapter 14
Chronic Illness

MARY S. NICHOLS

CHAPTER OBJECTIVES

After studying this chapter, the student should be able to:

- Differentiate between acute and chronic illness.
- Describe factors that influence chronic illness.
- Identify areas of assessment of the chronically ill person.
- Describe physical and psychosocial interventions for chronic illness.
- Define rehabilitation and the roles of team members (especially the nurse) and of the patient.
- Describe different patterns and facilities for continuing care.
- Identify major health goals related to chronic health problems to be achieved by 1990.

PREREQUISITE READING

Long-Phipps, Chapter 14, pp. 291-311.

SELF-ASSESSMENT ACTIVITIES

I. Define the following terms.

Ambulatory care
Compliance
Exacerbation
Natural history of disease
Noncompliance
Primary prevention
Rehabilitation
Remission
Respite care
Secondary prevention
Tertiary prevention

II. Discuss the following concepts.

1. Chronic disease is one of the major health problems in the United States.

2. As the population in this country ages, the incidence and prevalence of chronic disease can be expected to increase.

3. The Bureau of the Census estimates that there are 110 million persons with chronic disease in the United States.

4. Black Americans and other minorities have a higher incidence of health problems than do Caucasians.

5. Chronic illness characteristics include one or more of the following:
   a. Illness or permanent impairment

   b. Residual disability

   c. Nonreversible pathologic alterations that require long-term care

6. Chronic illnesses may be present at birth or develop over the lifespan.

7. Effective treatment prolongs the life of some children with chronic illnesses.

8. The rates for arthritis and hypertension are higher in black people than in white people.

9. Cultural values determine how nurses and patients view chronic illness.

10. Many persons with chronic illness will require financial assistance.

11. What are the reasons for noncompliance with the therapeutic recommendations?

12. The nurse's role requires involvement in prevention of chronic illnesses on three levels: primary, secondary, and tertiary. Discuss each level and list ideas you may develop.
    a. Primary

    b. Secondary

    c. Tertiary

III. Multiple choice

1. When caring for persons with a chronic illness in a long-term care setting, the nurse should:
   - **a.** Keep the patients in pajamas or a gown so that they will remember that they are ill
   - **b.** Anticipate the patients' needs and perform all activities for them because they are ill
   - **c.** Focus on strengthening the patients' capabilities rather than their disabilities
   - **d.** Help the patients remember that they have a chronic illness for which there is no cure
2. The person who is ultimately responsible for achieving the goals of rehabilitation is the:
   - **a.** Nurse
   - **b.** Doctor
   - **c.** Patient
   - **d.** Physical therapist
3. Which statement about home care is incorrect?
   - **a.** The primary providers of home care are nurses.
   - **b.** Home care is less costly than institutional care.
   - **c.** Home care is the best treatment setting for all patients with chronic illnesses.
   - **d.** Nursing care is the primary element of home care.

Mr. Zarcosky, age 50, has hypertension. He has been on antihypertensive medication and a weight reduction diet for 1 year. Mr. Zarcosky comes to the doctor's office for his routine check-up. Upon reviewing his medical record, the nurse finds that his blood pressure has been within normal range for the past year and that he has had no more complaints of headache.

4. According to these findings, his illness is in a state of:
   - **a.** Remission
   - **b.** Exacerbation

Two years later when he returns for his routine check-up Mr. Zarcosky's blood pressure is extremely elevated. When the nurse asks him what blood pressure medication he had been taking, he replies that he had stopped taking the medication even though he had been told that he would have to take it for his lifetime.

5. To plan ways to help him comply with the prescribed medication regimen, the nurse must first:
   - **a.** Warn him of the severe consequences for not following doctor's orders
   - **b.** Tell him that the doctor will stop seeing him if he does not take the medication as prescribed
   - **c.** Find out why he stopped taking the medication
   - **d.** Let him know that his current crisis is a punishment for not following doctor's orders

Mrs. Graham has a medical diagnosis of insulin-dependent diabetes mellitus. The present status indicates that she will always have to have dietary supervision, visit her physician, test her urine for the presence of glucose and acetone.

6. Persons with a chronic illness should be taught all of the following concepts *except:*
   - **a.** A chronic illness is one caused by disease that produces signs and symptoms
   - **b.** The disease runs a long course
   - **c.** Only partial recovery can be expected
   - **d.** Their disease was acute when it began
7. Mrs. Graham will be taught that she may *not* expect with medical supervision:
   - **a.** To be able to help prevent medical crisis
   - **b.** To be able to control symptoms by following a prescribed regimen
   - **c.** That payment will be arranged for treatment
   - **d.** To maintain normal interactions with others
8. The diagnostic title the nurse may select for Mrs. Graham is most likely to be:
   - **a.** Knowledge deficit (specify)
   - **b.** Anxiety
   - **c.** Potential for injury: trauma
   - **d.** Impaired skin integrity

Mrs. Weeks, a 77-year-old widow, was found on the floor of her mobile home by her next-door neighbor. She was transported to the hospital where a diagnosis of stroke was made. She has right-sided paralysis and slurred speech.

9. Rehabilitation for Mrs. Weeks will begin:
- **a.** On hospital admission
- **b.** A few days before discharge from the hospital
- **c.** When referral is made to a rehabilitation center
- **d.** When it is requested by the patient

The next-door neighbor informs the nurse that Mrs. Weeks lives alone but has two daughters. Her older daughter has consented to have Mrs. Weeks live with her when she is ready to be discharged from the hospital.

10. The nurse can help the daughter to care for Mrs. Weeks at home by doing all of the following *except:*
- **a.** Offering to provide a loan to help cover her medical expenses
- **b.** Teaching the daughter about Mrs. Weeks's illness and the type of care she will require
- **c.** Providing the daughter with a list of support agencies and organizations within the community
- **d.** Providing opportunities for the family to vent their feelings and anxieties

11. The most significant outcome of chronic illness that Mrs. Weeks and her family will experience will be:
- **a.** Fear
- **b.** Nutritional deficits
- **c.** Depersonalization
- **d.** Loss

IV. Write your answers in the space provided.

1. List four chronic illnesses.

2. List at least six reasons that patients may be noncompliant with prescribed medical regimens.

3. Why is it difficult to do epidemiologic studies of chronic illnesses?

4. Why is it important to study the natural history of a disease?

CLINICAL ACTIVITIES

1. Visit a rehabilitation center to find out what assessment tools are used to assess the needs and capabilities of chronically ill persons. What types of chronic illness are served by the center?
2. Is there a rehabilitation program for cardiac patients and patients with chronic pulmonary disorders in your community?

SUGGESTED READINGS

Bennett, HL: Why patients don't follow instructions, RN 49:45-47, Mar 1986.

How to use the skill of communication and negotiation to get a noncompliant patient to follow the treatment program.

Feldman, KF: Respite care: what nurses need to know, Home Health Care Nurs 4:35-43, July/Aug 1986.

Defines respite care, who funds it, and who uses it. Identifies sources of respite care services. Describes the caregivers and their special problems. Explains pros and cons of hospital-based programs and day care programs.

Piano, LA: Adult day care: A new ambulatory care alternative, Nursing 16:60-63, Aug 1986.

Through use of a case study, the author describes criteria for screening candidates, use of a multidisciplinary approach, the importance of family involvement, and what a typical day at a center may consist of.

Tydell, P: Are there opportunities in your own backyard? Nursing 87 17:77, June 1987.

Williams, SR: Nutrition in rehabilitation. In Nutrition and diet therapy, St Louis, 1985. The CV Mosby Co.

Chapter 15

Dying, Death, and Loss

VIVIENNE I. WALTON

CHAPTER OBJECTIVES

On completion of this chapter, the student shoud be able to:

- Differentiate among dying, death, and loss; define clinical death.
- Identify some rights of dying persons and describe a "living will."
- How do autonomy, informed consent, and paternalism relate to quality of life for the dying person?
- Describe four attitudinal dimensions of death: denial, defiance, desire, and acceptance.
- Describe the stages/phases of dying proposed by Kubler-Ross, Pattison, and Martocchio.
- Describe effects on the family when a family member dies.
- Differentiate among grief, bereavement, and mourning, and describe the grief syndrome.
- Identify assessment parameters for the dying person.
- Describe general nursing interventions for grievers and the dying person.

PREREQUISITE READING

Long-Phipps, Chapter 15, pp. 313-328.

SELF-ASSESSMENT ACTIVITIES

I. Define the following terms.

Active euthanasia
Autonomy
Bereavement
Brain death
Clinical death
Commission
Confidant
Death
Death with dignity
Dying
Descending plateaus
Downward slopes
Ethics
Euthanasia
Gradual slants
Grief
Grief syndrome
Informed choice
Informed consent
Living will
Loss
Mental capacity
Mourning
Omission
Passive euthanasia
Paternalism
Peaks and valleys
Principle autonomy
Process of Grieving
Quality of life
Right to die
Searching behaviors
Voluntary euthanasia

II. For your consideration.

1. How would you interpret the following expressions as they relate to your death?
   a. Good death
   b. Death with dignity
   c. Dying is a part of living
   d. Dying well

2. What are your perceptions about your death? Do you view it as:
   a. Punishment
   b. Failure
   c. An achievement
   d. Something to look forward to
   e. Something to fear
   f. Something that's avoidable and unnecessary
   g. A way to achieve immortality
3. Would you make out a living will? Why or why not?

4. What are your beliefs about prolonging life by any means?

5. Why is it important for you as a nurse to view the dying process in terms of stages or phases?

6. Would you want to be told you are dying?

7. What would constitute quality of life for you if you were dying? Who determines what the quality of life is for you as a dying person?

8. What are your views on euthanasia?

III. Match the terms below with the appropriate theorists, using the initials shown below.

(K) Kübler-Ross's stages of dying
(M) Martocchio's patterns of living-dying
(P) Pattison's phases of dying

1. _____ Anger, bargaining, and denial
2. _____ Peaks and valleys
3. _____ Chronic living-dying
4. _____ Gradual slants
5. _____ Terminal
6. _____ Shock and disbelief
7. _____ Acute living-dying
8. _____ Depression and acceptance
9. _____ Descending plateaus
10. _____ Downward slopes

IV. Multiple choice

1. There is a movement to recognize that dying persons have rights. Which of the following is not considered a right?
   a. To know one is seriously ill and may die.
   b. To die in an atmosphere of hopefulness.
   c. To be cared for by people who are least knowledgeable.
   d. To die in peace and dignity.

2. Which of the following is not a prevailing societal attitude toward death?
   a. Death denial
   b. Desire for decision
   c. Death defiance
   d. Death acceptance
3. Which of the following is not a consideration in choosing to die at home?
   a. Observations of responses to interventions
   b. The desires of the dying person
   c. The resources (economic, psychologic, and physical) of the family members
   d. Careful planning, instruction, and support systems
4. The phases of grief syndrome are:
   a. Shock and disbelief
   b. Anger, disorganization, and despair
   c. Identification, reorganization, and restitution
   d. All of the above

V. Answer the following items as true (T) or false (F).

1. _____ Living wills are legally enforceable in all states.
2. _____ The expectations of living have changed as life expectancies have changed.
3. _____ Both dying and death have unique aspects that evoke fear, anxieties, and uncertainties.
4. _____ Informed consent assumes that the person lacks the ability to understand, process data, and make decisions.
5. _____ Paternalism is the ability to accept or acquiesce to another person's wishes, choices, or actions for that person's own benefit.
6. _____ Living-dying are opposite ends of a continuum.
7. _____ Dying persons do not confide in every nurse.
8. _____ The experience of dying may serve as a cohesive force in some families and a disruptive force in others.
9. _____ Timing of the sharing of information and the type and amount of information given at any one session are irrelevant.
10. _____ Peer support is most beneficial to nurses caring for dying persons.

VI. Write your answers in the spaces provided.

1. What are the nursing interventions for grievers?

2. What are the nursing interventions for the dying person?

3. Complete a nursing assessment of mental capacity.

4. What are the nursing evaluation methods in the care of the dying patient and significant others?

CASE STUDY

Nikki Hopcroft, age 36, comes to the hospital for a left breast biopsy with possible modified radical mastectomy. When she had her annual physical examination 2 days ago, the doctor discovered a large, hard, nonpliable lump in her left breast and recommended hospitalization for a biopsy. At that time, the doctor also informed her that there was a strong possibility that the lump was cancerous.

The day after her admission to the hospital, Mrs. Hopcroft goes to surgery; a left modified radical mastectomy is performed. When Mrs. Hopcroft returns to the clinical unit and fully recovers from anesthesia, she looks at and feels the site of her left breast to discover that it is covered with a large, tight dressing. She also discovers that it is painful to move her left arm, which is elevated on a pillow. A Hemovac drain is in place and connected on a pillow. A Hemovac drain is in place and connected to continuous wall suction.

When the nurse enters to check Mrs. Hopcroft's condition, she finds her crying. When the nurse asks if anything is troubling her, Mrs. Hopcrift shakes her head negatively and says, "Oh, my arm's just a little sore when I try to move it."

Later, the doctor visits to tell her the results of the biopsy and explain plans for follow-up treatment. In his explanation, when he comes to the word biopsy, Mrs. Hopcroft suddenly interrupts him. She throws up her right hand and says in a sobering tone, "Stop! Stop! I don't want to hear it. I just want some peace for just a moment. Go ahead and do whatever you want to do with me."

"I can understand how you feel, Mrs. Hopcroft," says the doctor. He continues, "You are going to need chemotherapy. Dr. Jason, who is an oncologist, will be by tomorrow to talk with you about it and to set up a follow-up schedule for treatment later."

A total body scan is performed and reveals metastasis to the lungs. However, Mrs. Hopcroft continues to request that she not be told the test results, while consenting to any treatment.

1. What phase of the grief process is Mrs. Hopcroft experiencing?
2. As confidant, what would be appropriate nursing actions?
3. Should the doctor have told Mrs. Hopcroft the test results even though she expressed a strong desire not to be informed of the results? Give a reason for your answer.

Nineteen months later, Mrs. Hopcroft's condition begins to deteriorate rapidly, and she is hospitalized for severe dyspnea. She now requires oxygen continuously. She is extremely weak and requires total care. Seeing that his wife is dying, Mr. Hopcroft decides to care for her at home.

4. What factors should be considered in planning home care for Mrs. Hopcroft?

Four months later, the nurse who took care of Mrs. Hopcroft happens to see Mr. Hopcroft at the grocery store. When the nurse inquires about Mrs. Hopcroft, he informs her that his wife died 3 weeks ago.

5. What questions could the nurse ask to assess where Mr. Hopcroft is in the grief process?
6. The nurse knows that there are many factors that affect a survivor's response to death. What are they?

SUGGESTED READINGS

Archer, DN and others: Sorrow has many faces: helping families cope with grief, Nurs 88 18(5): 43-45, 1988.

Clough, JG: Making life and death decisions you can live with, RN 51(5): 28-30, 1988.

Darden, J: Dying at home, AD Nurse 3(1): 21-22, 1988.

Featherstone, RG: Care of the sudden death survivors: the aberrant cardiac patients, Heart Lung 17(3): 242-246, 1988.

Jezurski, MB: We hurt too. . . nurses do experience pain, Nurs 88 18(4):160, 1988.

Mauritzen, J: Pastoral care for the dying and bereaved, Death Studies 12(2): 111-122, 1988.

Muller, JH and others: When is a patient "dying"? Calif Nurse 8(5): 4-5, 1988.

Serdahely, W and others: What carers need to understand about the near-death experience. Geriatr Nurs 9(4): 238-241, 1988.

Wilson, C: Psychological aspects of physical illness: comforting the newly bereaved. Nurs Time 83(48): 40-42, 1987.

Zambelli, GC and others: An interdisciplinary approach to clinical intervention for childhood bereavement, Death Studies 12(1): 41-50, 1988.

UNIT IV Perioperative Nursing

Chapter 16

Preoperative Nursing

JACQUELINE S. SPRAGUE

CHAPTER OBJECTIVES

On completion of this chapter, the student should be able to:

- Describe different purposes of surgery.
- Identify psychologic and physiologic responses to surgery.
- Identify risk factors for surgery.
- Explain the nature of informed consent and related nursing responsibilities.
- Explain the rationale for collection of physiologic data for the preoperative patient.
- Explain the preoperative preparation of the patient (diet, bowel and skin preparation).
- Identify common learning needs of preoperative patients and methods for deep breathing and coughing and leg exercises.
- Explain final preparation of the patient for surgery.

PREREQUISITE READING

Long-Phipps, Chapter 16, pp. 329-346.

SELF-ASSESSMENT ACTIVITIES

I. Define the following terms.

Ambulatory surgery
Anxiety
Deep breathing and coughing exercises
Informed consent
Major surgery
Postoperative leg exercises
Preanesthetic medications
Preoperative check list
Preoperative phase
Psychologic preparation

II. Multiple choice

1. The nurse's responsibility when caring for a patient experiencing surgery is to assist the patient:
   a. To cope with stressors
   b. To seek relief from pain
   c. To return to optimal functioning
   d. All of the above
2. Removal of a diseased gallbladder is an example of which type of surgery?
   a. Palliative
   b. Restorative
   c. Curative
   d. Diagnostic

3. An example of a neuroendocrine response to surgery would be:
   a. Increased GI motility
   b. Vasodilation
   c. Potassium retention
   d. Sodium retention
4. The most common fear experienced by patients undergoing surgery is:
   a. Fear of pain
   b. Fear of dying
   c. Fear of loss of control
   d. Fear of the unknown
5. Legal responsibility for obtaining informed consent from the patient resides with:
   a. The physician
   b. The nurse
   c. The admissions officer
   d. The anesthetist
6. Obesity predisposes the surgical patient to all of the following postoperative complications *except:*
   a. Electrolyte imbalance
   b. Wound dehiscence
   c. Respiratory problems
   d. Thrombophlebitis
7. The effect of moderate to severe anxiety on patients preoperatively:
   a. Enhances learning of postoperative procedures taught
   b. Decreases ability to cope with surgery
   c. Decreases possibility of complications in the postoperative period
   d. Decreases amount of preanesthetic medication needed
8. Mr. Grant is scheduled for surgery (a bowel resection). The evening before his surgery, he is visiting in other patients' rooms, talking incessantly, and telling jokes to the nurses. He will not sit down and rest more than a few minutes at a time. What should his assigned nurse's response be to this behavior?
   a. Contact the doctor for an order for a tranquilizer.
   b. Talk with Mr. Grant to determine the cause of his anxiety.
   c. Ignore his actions because this is normal preoperative behavior.
   d. Call his wife to come in and keep him company.
9. During the preoperative period, the patient's metabolism is:
   a. Decreased
   b. Increased
   c. Unchanged
   d. Dependent on his sex
10. Preanesthetic medications are given to:
   a. Allow for a smoother induction and maintenance of anesthesia
   b. Decrease salivary and respiratory secretions
   c. Decrease anxiety
   d. All of the above

III. Match the terms with the appropriate definitions.

a. Abdomen rises and falls
b. Final preparation for surgery
c. Press back of knee against bed, lift heel
d. For healthy persons requiring uncomplicated surgery
e. Given for GI, pelvic, perianal surgeries
f. Avoid venous stasis
g. Decreases microorganisms at operative site

1. _____ Skin preparation
2. _____ Quadriceps drill
3. _____ Diaphragmatic breathing
4. _____ Postoperative leg exercises
5. _____ Preoperative check list
6. _____ Ambulatory surgery
7. _____ Enema

IV. Complete the following teaching plan.

Assessment	Nursing diagnosis	Goals	Intervention	Evaluation
Patient is scheduled for a partial gastrectomy in 2 days. When asked if she knew what exercises to perform postoperatively to enhance her recovery, she replied, "No, I don't."	Knowledge deficit related to turning, coughing, deep breathing, and leg exercises postoperatively			

V. Complete the crossword puzzle.

ACROSS

1. Suffix for removal of an organ or gland
2. Suffix for suturing or stitching
3. Type of surgery done to relieve symptoms without curing disease
4. Type of surgery done to determine cause of symptoms
5. Suffix which means providing an opening

DOWN

5. Suffix which means cutting into
6. Type of surgery done to strengthen a weakened area
7. Type of surgery done to remove a diseased part
8. Suffix which means looking into
9. Suffix which means plastic repair

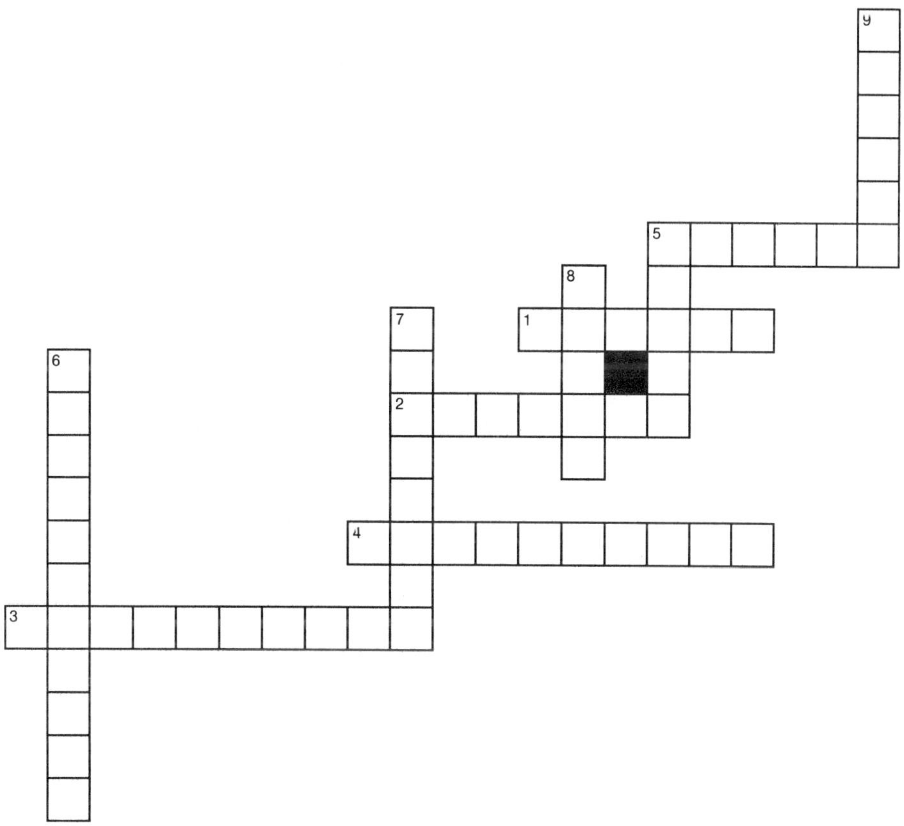

CASE STUDY

Mrs. Jaimerson, a 64-year-old retired schoolteacher, has been admitted to the hospital with a diagnosis of gangrene of the left large toe. The left large toe is dry, wrinkled, and black. Her left foot is cool to touch, with slow capillary refill. Her left foot becomes darkened in color when she holds it in a dependent position, but the right foot remains normal in color. Circulation in the right foot is adequate. It is warm to touch and has good capillary refill. The pedal pulse in the left foot is nonpalpable, but strong in the right foot. The femoral pulses are pesent and equal.

This morning she is complaining of pain in the left foot and states that the pain is less severe when she sits on the side of the bed. She is scheduled for whirlpool of the left foot at 10 AM. She has an IV of D^5W with 5% alcohol infusing in the left forearm via IVAC at 50 ml/hr. The IV site shows no signs of infiltration.

When the nurse enters her room with the wheelchair to transport her to physical therapy for whirlpool, she states that the doctor told her that the only alternative remaining is to amputate her left foot just above the ankle. She begins to cry and says, "I'm afraid I won't be any good after they take off my foot. I might as well be dead."

The physician's progress notes reveal that surgery is scheduled in 2 days.

1. Formulate a nursing diagnosis for each patient problem described in the case study. You should have at least three.
2. What would be the appropriate response for the nurse to make to Mrs. Jaimerson's statements?
3. With one student acting as the nurse and one as the patient, role-play the above case study to demonstrate how to assess the patient's preoperative teaching-learning needs and how to intervene to meet those needs.

DIRECTIONS FOR RESEARCH

The primary purpose of splinting an incision is to reduce pain when coughing. Patients have traditionally been taught to splint by several methods: with a pillow, with a towel, or with the hands. Perform an informal survey on your patient to determine which method of splinting most effectively reduces incisional pain when coughing.

CLINICAL ACTIVITIES

1. Examine the preoperative checklist at your clinical agency and identify the routine preoperative screening tests required for surgical patients. How current must each test be?
2. Prepare an assigned patient for surgery by using the preoperative checklist provided by your clinical agency and the Quick-Check Preoperative Assessment Guide in this study guide. The Quick-Check Preoperative Assessment Guide is designed to be used in conjunction with the agency's preoperative checklist. Use of the two forms together will ensure comprehensive, individualized preoperative care of the surgical patient.
3. Talk with surgical patients (include preoperative and postoperative patients) to find out what their greatest source of anxiety was about the surgical experience. Also, find out what they did or what another health worker did that was most helpful to them in resolving their preoperative anxiety.
4. Examine your clinical agency's policy regarding informed consent and the nurse's role in the informed consent process. Discuss findings in clinical post conference.

QUICK-CHECK PREOPERATIVE ASSESSMENT GUIDE	Yes	No
1. Is the hospital's preop checklist completed?		
If YES is checked for any of the following areas below, describe in the nurses notes.		
2. Is patient experiencing alterations in the following: **a.** Sensory functioning (i.e., vision, hearing, parasthesia, etc.)		
b. Motor functioning (i.e., weakness, paralysis, etc.)		
c. Nutritional status (i.e., anorexia, nausea, vomiting)		
d. Bowel elimination (i.e., diarrhea, constipation)		
e. Urinary elimination (voiding problems)		
f. Comfort (i.e., pain, insomnia, numbness)		
3. Does patient have any intrusive devices (IVs, Foley, oxygen, N/G tube, etc.)?		
4. Are instrusive devices functioning properly?		
5. Does patient have any prosthetic devices in place which will be left in place (i.e., eyes, hearing aids, cardiac pacemaker, joint implants)?		
6. Has chart been flagged to alert OR personnel of any prosthetic devices?		
7. Does patient know: **a.** How to perform coughing and deep breathing exercises?		
b. How to turn in bed?		
c. How to perform bed exercises?		
d. Purpose of a, b, and c?		
e. In general terms, what to expect preoperatively and postoperatively?		
8. Has patient been given an opportunity to ventilate concerns or anxieties about surgery or anesthesia?		

Check each assessment area and record findings in nurse's notes

A. Bowel sounds: present _____ absent _____ hypoactive _____ hyperactive _____
B. Status of abdomen: soft _____ nontender _____
distended _____ other (describe) __________________________
C. Peripheral pulses: present _____ equal _____
nonpalpable _____ other (describe) __________________________
D. Color of skin and nailbeds: WNL _____ other (describe) __________________________
E. Breath sounds: clear _____ abnormal (describe) __________________________
F. Level of consciousness: alert oriented _____
semicomatose _____ comatose _____
confused _____ disoriented _____
lethargic _____ stuporous _____
G. Capillary refill: Upper extremities adequate _____ poor _____
Lower extremities adequate _____ poor _____
H. General condition of skin: dry _____ edema (describe) __________________________
warm _____ other (describe) __________________________
I. Neck vein distention: present _____ absent _____
J. Heart Sounds: WNL _____ other (describe) __________________________
If Patient is to have urologic surgery, in addition to the above, check:
K. Color of urine: yellow _____ clear _____ amber _____
other (describe) __________________________
If Patient to have neurological surgery, in addition to the above check:
L. Pupillary reaction: PERRLA _____ other (describe) __________________________
M. Hand grips: strong _____ equal _____ other (describe) __________________________

SUGGESTED READINGS

Gamotis, P, and others: Inpatient vs outpatient satisfaction: a research study, AORN J 47(6):00, 1988.
Moss, V: Music and the surgical patient, AORN J 48(1):64-69, 1988.
Reasearch article on therapeutic effect of music on perioperative patients' anxiety level, with implications for nursing.

Chapter 17

Intraoperative Intervention

BRENDA GOODNER

CHAPTER OBJECTIVES

On completion of this chapter, the student should be able to:

- Explain the concept of perioperative nursing care.
- Identify the members of the surgical team and describe their individual responsibilities.
- Identify the basic rules of surgical asepsis.
- Explain the rationale for operating room attire and personnel health habits.
- Identify factors that promote patient safety in the operating room.
- Describe five common positions for patients undergoing surgery and specify the nursing care planning involved.
- Describe the various methods of administering anesthetics and identify the common agents used for each.
- Identify the various methods available for monitoring patients during surgical procedures.
- Describe nursing interventions to ensure safe patient care when the surgical procedure has been completed and before transfer to the recovery area.

PREREQUISITE READING

Long-Phipps, Chapter 17, pp. 347-369.

SELF-ASSESSMENT ACTIVITIES

I. Define the following terms.

Aseptic technique
Association of Operating Room Nurse (AORN)
Circulating nurse
Dissociative anesthesia
General anesthetic
Gowning and gloving
Hypothermia
Intraoperative phase
Local anesthetic
Malignant hyperthermia
Perioperative nursing
Postoperative phase
Preoperative phase
Regional anesthetic
Scrub nurse
Surgical asepsis

II. Answer the following questions.

1. What is the intraoperative phase of surgery?

2. What are nursing responsibilities during the intraoperative phase in the following areas?

a. Maintenance of safety
b. Physiological monitoring
c. Psychological monitoring

3. The scrubbed sterile members of the operating team are:

4. The nonsterile members of the operating team are:

5. What are the major responsibilities of the scrub nurse?

6. What are the major responsibilities of the circulating nurse?

7. Discuss the following four stages of anesthesia.
   Stage I

   Stage II

   Stage III

   Stage IV

8. What are the signs of toxicity to local anesthetics?

9. Discuss the guidelines for surgical scrub.

III. Match the following positions with the appropriate description.

a. Patient lies on side
b. Patient lies on back with buttocks to edge of table; thighs and legs are placed in stirrups
c. Patient lies on abdomen with face turned to one side, arms at side, palms pronated
d. Head and body are lowered into a head-down position and held in place with padded shoulder braces
e. Head is elevated and feet are lowered
f. Flat on back with arms at side, palms down, legs straight

1. _____ Supine
2. _____ Prone
3. _____ Trendelenburg
4. _____ Reverse Trendelenburg
5. _____ Lithotomy
6. _____ Lateral

IV. Multiple choice

1. The operative phase in which the nurse assures that the sponge and instrument counts are correct is the:
   a. Perioperative phase
   b. Preoperative phase
   c. Intraoperative phase
   d. Postoperative phase

2. In the operating room there are two categories of personnel—scrubbed sterile and nonsterile. Of those listed, who is the nonsterile member?
   a. Surgeon's assistant
   b. Circulating nurse
   c. Scrub nurse
   d. Primary physician
3. Patients are returned slowly from the operative position to the supine position to prevent what condition or effect?
   a. Injury to muscles
   b. Sudden drop in blood pressure
   c. Respiratory distress
   d. Discomfort
4. Two of the most common postoperative problems associated with the use of general anesthesia are:
   a. Seizures and bradycardia
   b. Muscle rigidity and hypertension
   c. Respiratory depression and hypotension
   d. Hemorrhage and depressed respirations
5. Nonintrusive hypothermia is most often obtained by what method?
   a. Extracorporeal cooling
   b. Cooling blankets
   c. Immersion in ice water
   d. Application of ice
6. Epinephrine is added to local anesthetics to:
   a. Initiate vasoconstriction
   b. Produce vasodilation
   c. Prevent vasospasm
   d. Increase blood pressure
7. The nurse planning the care of the patient undergoing spinal anesthesia must include adequate fluid intake. The reason for this is:
   a. To prevent dehydration
   b. To prevent postoperative headache
   c. To replace lost spinal fluid
   d. To enhance urinary output
8. The surgeon is ready to begin the operation when the patient enters which stage of anesthesia?
   a. I
   b. II
   c. III
   d. IV
9. The nurse should anticipate doing which of the following during the recovery period for the surgical patient who received Ketamine as an anesthetic?
   a. Checking pupillary reaction frequently
   b. Maintaining a quiet environment
   c. Keeping the patient in reverse Trendelenburg position
   d. Administering Dantrium to counteract the effects of anesthesia
10. A major postoperative problem associated with the use of muscle relaxants in combination with other anesthetics is:
   a. Mild seizures
   b. Acute urinary retention
   c. Hemorrhage
   d. Respiratory depression

11. To ensure that the patient has been safely and properly positioned on the OR table, the nurse should check to be sure that:
    - **a.** The operative site is easily accessible to the surgeon even though the body is not in good alignment
    - **b.** Bony prominences have been padded to reduce pressure
    - **c.** Sterile drapes are applied around the operative site only and the remainder of the body left exposed to allow circulation to be checked
    - **d.** No straps are applied to the extremities to prevent self-injury in the event of a seizure
12. The type of position a patient is placed in during surgery is determined by:
    - **a.** The type of surgical procedure to be performed
    - **b.** The patient's level of anesthesia
    - **c.** The age of the patient
    - **d.** The anesthesiologist
13. The surgical scrub is done:
    - **a.** After donning the gown and gloves
    - **b.** After donning the mask and gown
    - **c.** Before donning the gown and gloves
    - **d.** Just before entering surgical suite

V. Discuss the seven basic rules of surgical asepsis.

SUGGESTED READINGS

Driscoll, J: Environmental control and safety in the OR, Today's OR Nurse 2:18-22, March 1980.

Describes an environmental control program including electrical safety, accident prevention aseptic practice, processing control of supplies and equipment, and decontamination procedures.

Kleinstuber, M: Holding area serving the surgical patient, Today's OR Nurs 2:11-17, June 1980.

Provides a physical description of the holding area, the functional objectives of the area nurse, job descriptions of the RN in charge, the nursing assistant, and the OR Nurse, and the doctor's role. Care of the surgical patient is explained. A preoperative and postoperative assessment guide is provided.

Chapter 18

Postoperative Intervention

JACQUELINE S. SPRAGUE

CHAPTER OBJECTIVES

On completion of this chapter, the student should be able to:

- Identify nursing interventions to meet patient needs in the postanesthetic period.
- Discuss the rationale for collection of data necessary to plan nursing care when the patient returns to the clinical unit.
- Describe the types and process of wound healing and interventions that promote wound healing.
- Explain wound dehiscence and evisceration and appropriate nursing interventions.
- Identify postoperative respiratory and circulatory problems, assessment parameters, and preventive measures.
- Describe possible postoperative problems with fluid and electrolyte balance, nutrition, elimination, and inactivity, and the assessment parameters and preventive measures.
- Describe measures to promote patients' physical and psychologic comfort in the post-operative period.

PREREQUISITE READING

Long-Phipps, Chapter 18, pp. 371-395.

SELF-ASSESSMENT ACTIVITIES

I. Define the following terms.

Atelectasis
Collagen
Dehiscence
Evisceration
Hemovac
Hypostatic pneumonia
Incentive spirometer
Paralytic ileus
Penrose drain
Pulmonary edema
TENS
Thrombophlebitis
Urinary retention
Wound healing by primary intention
Wound healing by secondary intention
Wound healing by tertiary intention

II. Fill in the blanks with the appropriate word(s).

1. In the immediate postoperative period, two of the most common causes of inadequate pulmonary exchange are ____________________ and ____________________.
2. Three causes of postoperative shock are:

   a. ____________________

   b. ____________________

   c. ____________________

3. Patients are discharged from the recovery room when the following criteria have been met:

   a. ____________________

   b. ____________________

   c. ____________________

4. List two safety measures to be taken to prevent injury to the patient in the immediate postoperative period:

   a. ____________________

   b. ____________________

   c. ____________________

5. Six parameters to be assessed on return of the surgical patient to the clinical unit are:

   a. ____________________ d. ____________________

   b. ____________________ e. ____________________

   c. ____________________ f. ____________________

III. Multiple choice

1. The postoperative patient's physical discomfort is focused on his or her:
   a. Incisional pain
   b. Fluid and electrolyte balance
   c. Emotional well-being
   d. Discharge from the recovery room
2. Which of the following is not a criterion for discharge from the recovery room?
   a. Vital signs are stable
   b. Decreased circulatory function
   c. Adequate respirations
   d. Returned motor function of anesthetized areas

Mr. Gower has returned to his clinical unit from the recovery room following a cholecystectomy. His wife and daughter have been visited and reassured by the surgeon. Mrs. Gower asks the nurse to explain her husband's condition.

3. The nurse's first reply to this request should be:
   a. "Mr. Gower is very comfortable following his abdominal surgery."
   b. "Tell me what Mr. Gower's surgeon has told you about his condition."
   c. "You are worried about your husband?"
   d. "Mr. Gower has been medicated for pain in the recovery room."
4. Indicate the assessment the nurse should make *first:*
   a. Safety
   b. Neurologic status
   c. Dressing
   d. Respiratory status
5. The nurse decides that Mr. Gower's respiratory status is adequate *when:*
   a. He uses only his abdominal muscles to exhale
   b. His respiratory rate is above 22/min
   c. His breathing is quiet and even
   d. His nostrils are flaring

6. Although Mr. Gower is still drowsy, to prevent postoperative pulmonary complications the nurse begins measures that would include:
   a. Massaging bony prominences
   b. Placing him in a high Fowler's position every 2 hours
   c. Encouraging a liberal fluid intake, orally
   d. Having him take a deep breath and cough every 2 hours
7. Mr. Gower's nurse knows that the clinical manifestations of shock include all *except:*
   a. A fall in blood pressure
   b. A decreased urinary output
   c. A weak, rapid, thready pulse
   d. Warm, moist skin
8. An early sign of shock is:
   a. Loss of consciousness
   b. Restlessness
   c. Decrease in blood pressure
   d. Cool skin
9. Mr. Gower's dressing is dry on the top. The nurse can assume that:
   a. There is no excessive bleeding in the incision
   b. She should check the side of the dressing for drainage
   c. He has no incisional drain
   d. The dressing is not too tight
10. Following general anesthesia, Mr. Gower's most comfortable position is *probably:*
   a. High Fowler's
   b. Head of bed slightly elevated
   c. Flat
   d. Sim's position
11. Mr. Gower's IV line is running at 25 ml/min on his return to his clinical unit. The most appropriate action for the nurse is to *first:*
   a. Slow the IV to 3 ml/min
   b. Notify the surgeon
   c. Check the IV order for correct rate
   d. Discontinue the IV immediately
12. The correct drainage system for a sump nasogastric tube is:
   a. Constant low electric suction
   b. Intermittent low electric suction
   c. Low negative pressure
   d. Gravity drainage
13. Which of the following areas of the medical record is *least* important for the nurse to check initially upon Mr. Gower's return from the recovery room?
   a. Physician's order sheet
   b. Hospital admission record
   c. Recovery room record
   d. Surgical notes
14. Which of the following is an intrinsic risk factor for postoperative thrombophelitis?
   a. Hip surgery
   b. Tight cast or dressing
   c. Shock
   d. Malnutrition
15. Monitoring for fluid overload is an important assessment activity postoperatively. Which of the following indicates fluid overload?
   a. Weight loss
   b. Cold, dry skin
   c. Moist breath sounds
   d. Excess appetite

16. To achieve the goal of reversing a nursing diagnosis of Altered Nutrition: Less than Body Requirements, the nurse should:
    - a. Encourage postoperative patients to eat foods high in vitamin D
    - b. Encourage bed rest while the patient is anorexic
    - c. Force food if the patient is anorexic
    - d. Help the patient with his plans for obtaining desired nutrients
17. Mr. Gower's incision has healed very well and he is ready for discharge. He still has some fatigue. This outcome is:
    - a. Not expected
    - b. Expected
18. A wound is sutured closed several days after trauma. It should heal by:
    - a. Primary intention
    - b. Tertiary intention
    - c. Secondary intention
    - d. Further draining
19. Collagen is deposited and granulation tissue is formed. This phase of wound healing is called:
    - a. Phase III
    - b. Phase I
    - c. Phase II
    - d. Phase IV
20. A patients abdominal surgical wound dehisces. This means that:
    - a. There is partial to complete separation of wound edges.
    - b. There has been inadequate wound closure
    - c. Abdominal viscera protrudes through the wall
    - d. The wound will not heal well when it is resutured

CASE STUDY

Donna Bosler, age 48, is an obese diabetic who has just arrived in the recovery room following a total abdominal hysterectomy. She remains unconscious and does not respond to verbal command. She has an IV of D-5/0.9% NS infusing into the left hand at 125 ml/hr. After 90 minutes, the nurse determines that Ms. Bosler is ready to be transferred to her assigned clinical unit. The recovery room nurse notifies the nurse on the clinical unit that Ms. Bosler will be brought back to her room in about 15 minutes.

Ms. Bosler arrives on the clinical unit and is safely transferred to her bed. She remains asleep, but arouses easily. When aroused, she is still very drowsy. The recovery room nurse reports that the incision was closed with metal staples, that there is a Penrose drain in place, and that the dressing can be changed PRN.

The nurse observes that it has been 5 hours since Ms. Bosler's surgery, and that she has not voided. The nurse assesses Ms. Bosler for signs of urinary retention and finds none present.

On the third postoperative day, Ms. Bosler complains of increased pain in the operative site. She states, "It feels like something suddenly popped." The nurse removes the abdominal dressing to discover that the wound has dehisced.

Two weeks later, Ms. Bosler is ready for discharge. She will go home with an abdominal dressing in place. The doctor left orders for her to make an appointment for a follow-up visit in 4 days.

■ ■ ■

Complete the following nursing care plan. Prioritize *all* the nursing diagnoses.

Assessment	Nursing diagnosis	Goals	Interventions	Outcome criteria

CLINICAL ACTIVITIES

1. When assigned to the recovery room:
   a. Observe who accompanies the patient from the OR to the recovery room.
   b. Listen to the report given to the recovery room nurse by the person accompanying the patient from the OR. What information did the report contain?
   c. Observe the recovery room nurse in the process of admitting the patient to the recovery room. What actions did the nurse perform?
   d. What is included in a frequent assessment of the patient?
   e. Examine the nurse's notes to see what kind of data is charted.
   f. What criteria does the nurse use to determine that the patient is ready for discharge to an assigned clinical unit?
2. Prepare a room on your assigned clinical unit to receive a patient from the recovery room.
3. Perform an assessment of a postoperative patient who has just returned to your assigned clinical unit from the recovery room.
4. Examine a postoperative patient's chart and identify factors that predispose the patient to *postoperative complications.* Has the patient experienced any complications? If so, list them and the risk factors that may have contributed to their development.
5. Write a nursing care plan on this patient that can be used postoperatively in the clinical unit.

SUGGESTED READINGS

AORN J. Nursing Practices Committee: A model for perioperative nursing practice, AORN J 41:192-193, Jan 1985.
A chart listing examples of perioperative nursing practices during the pre-, intra-, and postoperative phase is provided. Important data that the OR nurse should include in a verbal report to the RR nurse is outlined.

Montanari, J: Documenting your postop assessment findings: a new form you can use, Nurs 85 15:31-35, Aug 1985.
Provided is a step-by-step process of transferring the patient from the RR to the clinical unit. Information that the RR nurse should include in a verbal report to the RN on the clinical unit is outlined. The author also explains how to establish assessment priorities and provides a Postop assessment form that can be used.

Borchlardt, AC: Guide to solving postanesthesia problems, 18(5):66-86, 1988.

Neuberger, GB and others: A new look at wound care, Nurs 85 15:34-42, Feb 1985.
Excellent reading. The authors cover the chain of an infection, preoperative and intraoperative skin preparation, and postoperative wound care involving dressings, drains, sutures, and wound cleansing agents, their advantages and disadvantages.

Review essential skills: wound care sterile dressing change, administration of nasal oxygen, insertion of oral airway, arrangement of nasogastric tube to suction, oropharyngeal suctioning, management of IV infusion. (See: Potter, PA, and Perry, AG: Fundamentals of Nursing, St. Louis, 1985, The C.V. Mosby Co.)

Rogers, AL and others: Malignant hyperthermia: a perioperative emergency—home study program, AORN J 41:369-374, 376-378, Feb 1985.
The authors cover the etiology, pathophysiology, clinical manifestations, treatment, prevention, and nursing considerations. Also provided is a short, multiple-choice exam to allow for self-evaluation of the content on malignant hyperthermia.

UNIT V Sensorimotor Problems

Chapter 19

The Patient with Neurologic Problems

MARY S. NICHOLS

CHAPTER OBJECTIVES

On completion of this chapter, the student should be able to:

- Explain the difference in types of neurons and how they transmit impulses.
- List the divisions of the central nervous system, peripheral nervous system, and the autonomic nervous system.
- List four physiologic changes in the nervous system that occur with aging.
- Explain three components of the neurological assessment.
- Explain the importance of primary, secondary, and tertiary prevention in problems of the nervous system.
- State five symptoms of increased intracranial pressure.
- List five nursing actions to decrease intracranial pressure.
- List two degenerative diseases and three infection-related diseases of the nervous system and explain the pathophysiology involved.
- Define cerebrovascular accident, cerebral thrombosis, cerebral embolism, transient ischemic attack, and cerebral hemorrhage.
- State two complications of brain surgery.

PREREQUISITE READING

Long-Phipps, Chapter 19, pp. 397-513.

SELF-ASSESSMENT ACTIVITIES

I. Define the following terms.

Adiadochokinesia
AIDS
Akinetic seizures
Aphasia
Apneic breathing
Apraxia
Arbovirus
Areflexia
Arousal
Ataxic breathing
Aura
Autonomic dysreflexia
Awareness
Babinski's sign
Brudzinski's sign
Carotid endarterectomy
Causalgia
Cheyne-Stokes respiration
Clonic contractions
Cluster breathing
Coma
Concussion
Confusion
Consciousness
Contusion
Craniotomy
CSF
CVA
Decerebrate posturing
Decorticate posturing
Delirium
Depressed breathing
Diplopia
Disorientation
Dysarthria
Eaton-Lambert syndrome
Epilepsy
Fasciculations
Flaccidity
Gasping breathing
Hallucination
ICP
Illusion

Continued

Kernig's sign
Locked-in state
Meninges
Myoclonic seizures
Neuralgia
Neuritis
Nystagmus
Obtunded
Oculocephalic reflex response
Paralysis
Parasthesia
Paresis
Postictal period
Proprioception
Romberg test
Status epilepticus
Stereognosia
Sterile abcess
Stroke in evolution
Stupor
TIA
Tonic contraction
Unconscious
Vegetative state

II. Write your answers in the space provided.

1. What are effectors? What are the two classes of effectors?

2. What four chemicals allow excitatory transmission at the synaptic junction? What two chemicals inhibit transmission of nerve impulses at the synaptic junction?

3. What is the function of the blood-brain barrier?

4. What is the function of cerebrospinal fluid? Where is it formed? How is it excreted from the brain?

5. How many pairs of cranial nerves are in the peripheral nervous system? How many pairs of spinal nerves are in the peripheral nervous system?

6. Where do the cranial nerves originate?

7. List four classes of drugs that should be restricted 24 to 48 hours before a myelogram when a water-based dye (Metrizamide) is used.

8. In what position should the patient be kept following a myelogram in which an oil-base dye (Pantopaque) is used? Why?

III. Match the components of the cerebral cortex with its function.

a. Frontal lobe **c.** Temporal lobe
b. Parietal lobe **d.** Occipital lobe

1. _____ Memory storage
2. _____ Visual center
3. _____ Conceptualization
4. _____ Ability to recognize body parts left versus right
5. _____ Ability to write words

IV. Circle the appropriate terms in the description below of how nerve impulses are transmitted in the nervous system.

The cell membrane of the neuron exhibits differential permeability in that it is permeable to (oxygen, carbon dioxide, proteins) and impermeable to (oxygen, carbon dioxide, proteins). The inside of the neuron contains a high concentration of (potassium, sodium), whereas the outside of the cell is high in (potassium, sodium). In a resting state, all neurons possess a potential for action and are said to be (depolarized, polarized). When a neuron is stimulated, there is a sudden movement of (potassium, sodium) to the inside of the cell membrane, thus creating a (negative, positive) state inside the cell, while (potassium, sodium) moves outside the cell, thus causing (depolarization, polarization). After the impulse passes through each segment of the neuron, (depolarization, repolarization) occurs in which active transport mechanisms move (potassium, sodium) back into the cell and (potassium, sodium) outside the cell, thus returning the membrane to its normal resting potential state.

V. Multiple choice

1. Which of the following is a function of an astrocyte?
- **a.** Supports structures of neurons
- **b.** Produces CSF
- **c.** Takes part in phagocytosis
- **d.** Produces lipid-protein complex that forms myelin sheaths

2. Dendrites receive information at sites called:
- **a.** Microglia
- **b.** Neurons
- **c.** Synapses
- **d.** Ependyma

3. Golgi type II cells are found in the:
- **a.** Cerebral cortex
- **b.** Cerebellum
- **c.** Axon
- **d.** Brain and spinal cord

4. An action potential will be propagated at a greater velocity when (NOTE: select two answers):
- **a.** The diameter of the axon is larger
- **b.** The impulse is in the myelinated portions of the neuron
- **c.** The diameter of the axon is smaller
- **d.** The impulse is in the unmyelinated portions of the neuron

5. The term *dorsal spinocerebellar* indicates that the tract ends in the:
- **a.** Cerebral cortex
- **b.** Thalamus
- **c.** Cerebellum
- **d.** Spinal cord

6. Which of the following does *not* occur when the parasympathetic system is stimulated?
- **a.** Heart rate decreases
- **b.** Bronchi constrict
- **c.** Pupils dilate
- **d.** GI peristalsis increases

7. Which of the following does *not* occur when the sympathetic system is stimulated?
   a. Blood vessels constrict
   b. Anal sphincter closes
   c. GI peristalsis decreases
   d. Bronchi constrict
8. When you are assessing an individual's sensory status, the person should:
   a. Keep his or her eyes closed during the testing
   b. Wear glasses if needed
   c. Not eat or drink anything the morning of the examination
   d. Empty his or her bladder before the examination
9. To examine the ocular fundus, the examiner:
   a. Uses a Snellen chart
   b. Uses an ophthalmoscope
   c. Directs a flashlight onto the eye and observes pupillary response
   d. Has the individual follow the examiner's finger movements with one eye closed
10. Preparation of the patient for an EEG includes:
   a. Keeping the patient NPO the evening preceding the procedure
   b. Informing the patient that scalp hair will be shaved where the electrodes are attached
   c. Informing the patient that the test is painless
   d. Informing the patient that a radiopaque dye will be given intravenously and x-ray film will be taken
11. Which of the following test results of cerebral spinal fluid indicates an abnormality?
   a. The presence of glucose
   b. The presence of protein
   c. The CSF appears cloudy
   d. The absence of lymphocytes
12. Preparation of the patient for a brain scan involves:
   a. Informing the patient that a radiopaque dye will be administered intravenously
   b. Keeping the patient NPO after midnight before the test
   c. Assessing the patient for allergy to iodine
   d. Informing the patient that a radioactive isotope will be administered intravenously

VI. Match the type of seizure with the correct description.

a. Petit mal c. Grand mal
b. Psychomotor d. Jacksonian

1. _____ Type of seizure that occurs during childhood and gradually resolves as the person gets older
2. _____ Type of seizure characterized by a sudden vacant facial expression with eyes focused straight ahead and with little to no tonic-clonic movements
3. _____ Type of seizure manifested by antisocial behavior, the appearance of intoxication, and autonomic complaints
4. _____ Type of seizure manifested by tonic contractions involving the extremities initially; may or may not be progressive
5. _____ Type of seizure manifested by tonic and clonic contractions and loss of consciousness

VII. Write the answers to the following questions in the space provided.

1. List the six clinical manifestations of a grand mal seizure in the order in which they commonly occur.

2. What causes the epileptic cry?

3. What diagnostic test is used to evaluate seizure activity?

4. List the observations that should be made about a person having a seizure.

5. Why is good oral care a MUST for patients receiving phenytoin (Dilantin)?

6. Why are there such a wide variety of signs and symptoms of multiple sclerosis compared with any other neurologic disease?

7. How is diplopia treated in patients with multiple sclerosis?

8. List five drugs that patients with myasthenia gravis should avoid. Why?

9. What are the three causes of CVA?

10. What is the relationship between TIA and stroke?

11. What are the two most common sources of arboviral infections of the CNS?

12. Why is isolation not necessary with encephalitis?

13. What are the three most common organisms that cause brain abscess?

14. What effect does spinal cord injury have on sexual functioning of the male and the female?

15. List the four most frequently encountered types of brain tumors.

16. What position should the patient be placed in after an infratentorial craniotomy?

17. What is the most prominent neurologic manifestation associated with AIDS?

VIII. Multiple choice

1. A patient is brought to the emergency room in status epilepticus. The most important nursing goal for this patient would be:
   a. Maintain adequate ventilation
   b. Provide adequate rest
   c. Prevent fluid and electolyte imbalance
   d. Provide sensory stimuli

Mr. Bear is admitted to your clinical unit with a history of seizures. When you enter the room to obtain vital signs you observe him having a grand mal seizure. His jaws are clenched and respirations are noisy. A tongue blade is taped to the wall above his bed.

2. You should:
   a. Manually restrain the patient's arms to prevent injury
   b. Pry the patient's jaws open to insert the tongue blade
   c. Observe the patient and use your hands to protect the head
   d. Notify the cardiopulmonary resuscitation team
3. Which of the following would be *least* important for the nurse to chart when charting his or her observations about Mr. Bear's seizure?
   a. Identification of the type of seizure
   b. Duration of the seizure
   c. A description of the seizure activity
   d. A description of the patient's behavior after the seizure
4. The major adverse effect common to all anti-convulsant drugs is (NOTE: Select two answers.):
   a. Hypotension
   b. Pancytopenia
   c. Ataxia
   d. Drowsiness
5. Individuals taking prescribed medication for a seizure disorder:
   a. Can never drive a car
   b. Should be encouraged to lead a normal life
   c. Must follow a special diet to control the seizure
   d. Should be instructed to take the medication only when they feel a seizure coming on
6. Which drug is *not* used in the treatment of Parkinson's disease?
   a. Artane
   b. Cogentin
   c. Temaril
   d. Levodopa

Molly Paterson, age 45, has been admitted with a diagnosis of subarachnoid hemorrhage secondary to an aneurysm.

7. On assessment of Molly, you would anticipate finding all of the following *except:*
   a. Headache
   b. Photophobia
   c. Nausea and vomiting
   d. Hypotension

8. The physician has prescribed an intravenous infusion of aminocaproic acid (Amicar) for Molly. Which of the following goals would reflect the desired therapeutic response of this drug?
   a. The patient will be free of infection.
   b. Urinary output will be increased.
   c. Intracranial bleeding will cease.
   d. Nausea and vomiting will cease.
9. Nursing care for Molly will include all of the following *except:*
   a. Keeping her on bedrest
   b. Keeping her flat in bed
   c. Administering stool softeners
   d. Keeping her room dark and quiet

In an attempt to control intracranial bleeding, the physician applied a Silverton clamp to Molly's left common carotid artery. Each day the physician gradually tightens the clamp.

10. The primary reason that the physician gradually seals off the carotid artery is to:
    a. Allow time for the development of collateral circulation
    b. Prevent increased intracranial pressure
    c. Prevent headache
    d. Prevent the need for further surgery
11. The nurse would release the clamp if Molly experienced:
    a. Weakness of facial muscles
    b. Diminished level of consciousness
    c. Right-sided weakness
    d. All of the above
12. Care of the patient following a supratentorial craniotomy would include:
    a. Keeping the patient flat in bed with a small pillow under the shoulders
    b. Keeping the neck hyperextended
    c. Encouraging coughing frequently
    d. Keeping the patient in a semi-Fowler's position
13. With an upper motor neuron bladder the:
    a. Reflex arc is not intact
    b. Patient experiences acute urinary retention
    c. Bladder empties automatically without control
    d. Bladder is hypotonic
14. Which statement about herpes zoster is incorrect?
    a. It is caused by the varicella virus.
    b. It is communicable in patients who have had chicken pox.
    c. It is characterized by a vesicular skin rash.
    d. The involved areas are painful.
15. When caring for a patient with herpes zoster, you should wear:
    a. Mask only
    b. Mask and gloves
    c. Gloves only
    d. Mask, gown, and gloves
16. The primary manifestations of a brain abscess include all *except:*
    a. Hypotension
    b. Headache
    c. Fever
    d. Altered mentation

IX. Complete the chart on autonomic dysreflexia.

	Autonomic dysreflexia
Clinical manifestations	
Causes	
Site of cord lesion commonly associated with	
Complications	
Treatment	

X. Match the disease with the underlying pathology.

a. Muscular dystrophy
b. Multiple sclerosis
c. Guillain-Barre´ syndrome
d. Myasthenia gravis
e. Parkinson's disease

1. ______ Alteration in the uptake of acetycholine at the muscle receptor site
2. ______ Progressive, diffuse, irregular gray patches of demyelination of white matter in the brain and spinal cord
3. ______ Degeneration of cells in substantia nigra causing a decrease in production of dopamine
4. ______ Acute cellular mediated demyelination of the peripheral nerves, resulting in progressive loss of motor function from the lower extremities and upward
5. ______ Initial muscle hypertrophy due to infiltration of the muscle by fat and fibrous tissue, then progressive atrophy of muscles

XI. Place the number of the statement that describes the test beneath the appropriate test listed on p. 101. The statement may be used more than once.

1. A test for meningeal irritation.
2. A test for stance and balance.
3. A test in which positive findings indicate upper motor neuron disease.
4. The test is performed with the patient standing, feet close together, with eyes open and then closed.
5. The test is performed with the patient in a recumbent position.
6. A positive test is present when there is spasm of the hamstring muscles with resistance to extension of the leg and with head and neck pain.
7. A positive test is present when the hips and legs flex involuntarily as the neck is passively flexed.
8. A positive test is present when the great toe flexes toward the knee with fanning of the other toes as pressure is applied to the plantar surface of the foot from the heel toward the toes.
9. A positive test is present when the person begins to sway and lose balance.

Brudzinski's sign **Romberg's sign**

Babinski's sign **Kernig's sign**

XII. Multiple choice

1. Preparation of the patient for a nuclear magnetic resonance scan would involve all of the following *except:*
   a. Checking for the presence of metal prostheses or implants
   b. Informing the patient that the procedure is painless
   c. Informing the patient that a radioactive isotope will be given intravenously
   d. Informing the patient that the procedure is noisy
2. To assess orientation, the nurse would ask the patient to do all of the following *except:*
   a. State name
   b. Identify location
   c. State the answer to a simple math problem
   d. State the day, month, or year

Mr. Woods has a long history of chronic low-back pain. He is scheduled for a myelogram in which Metrizamide (a water-based dye) will be used.

3. Before the test is done, the nurse should do all of the following *except:*
   a. Check strength and seansation of his lower extremities
   b. Have him sign a permit for the procedure
   c. Inform him that he will be placed in several different positions as x-rays are taken
   d. Inform him that headaches do not occur with the use of water-base dyes
4. Care of Mr. Woods after the myelogram would include:
   a. Keeping him flat in bed for at least 24 hours
   b. Restricting fluid intake
   c. Assessing strength and sensation of the lower extremities
   d. Assisting him to ambulate once general anesthesia wears off
5. Which of the following structures of the cerebrum is responsible for postural adjustments and gross volitional movements?
   a. Pons
   b. Basal ganglia
   c. Medulla
   d. Thalamus
6. A patient is scheduled for an EMG. Which of the following statements would be *incorrect* when explaining this procedure to the patient?
   a. The test is done to assess electrical activity of the brain.
   b. Electrodes will be inserted into a muscle through which a small electrical current will pass.
   c. You will experience some discomfort with this procedure.
   d. Medication will be available after the procedure to relieve your discomfort.
7. Which of the following statements about the digital subtraction angiography is incorrect?
   a. A radiopaque dye is injected into an artery in the arm.
   b. The patient must sign a permit for the procedure.
   c. There are no activity restrictions after the procedure.
   d. The patient will be kept NPO the evening of the test.
8. When a radiopaque dye is used in diagnostic testing, the most important nursing assessment to make before the test is:
   a. Level of consciousness
   b. Allergy to iodine
   c. Status of the lungs
   d. Heart rate and rhythm

9. A patient is scheduled for a cerebral arteriogram. Before the test, the nurse marks an *X* over the pedal pulses of both of the patient's feet. The primary reason for this action is to:
   a. Aid the technician in determining where to insert the catheter to inject the dye
   b. Give the patient something to focus on while the test is being done
   c. Let the technician know that the feet are not to be used for vascular access
   d. Provide easy location of the pulses after the procedure
10. A patient returns to your clinical unit following a cerebral arteriogram in which the right femoral artery was used to inject the dye. A pressure dressing is in place at the right groin. Care of the patient would include:
   a. Encouraging ambulation to prevent thrombus formation
   b. Restricting fluid intake until general anesthetic wears off
   c. Keeping the patient on bedrest for overnight
   d. Removing the pressure dressing to prevent circulatory impairment

XIII. On performing a fundoscopic examination of a patient, you observe the following structures reflected in the figure below. Use the words below to label the structures.

Optic disk	Physiologic cup
Venule	Arteriole
Macular area	Fovea centralis

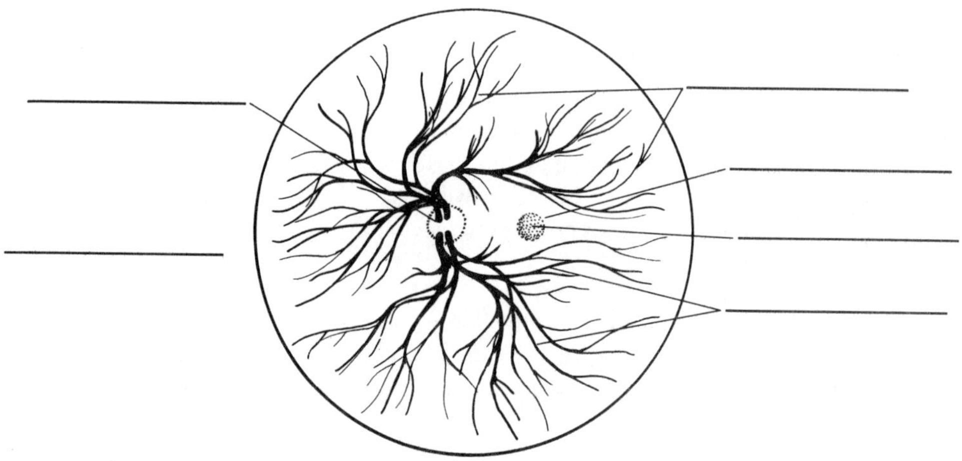

XIV. Write the appropriate term in the blank space to complete each sentence.

1. The type of aphasia in which comprehension of both written and spoken language is impaired is called ____________________.
2. The type of aphasia in which the person cannot comprehend what he hears or reads nor can he communicate his thoughts in writing or speech is called ____________________.
3. A person who has paralysis of both lower extremities is called a ____________________.
4. Drooping of the eyelids is called ____________________.
5. Swelling of the optic disc is called ____________________.
6. The space between the arachnoid mater and the pia mater is called the ____________________ space.
7. The outer layer of the meninges is called the ____________________ mater.
8. The term that means inequality of pupil size is ____________________.
9. The term that means lack of coordination of muscular movement is called ____________________.

XV. Write the name of the cranial nerve that corresponds with the roman numeral in the chart below. Then write the techniques you would use to assess functioning for each cranial nerve.

Nerve	Name	Assessments
I		
II		
III		
IV		
V		
VI		
VII		
VIII		
IX		
X		
XI		
XII		

XVI. Use the following terms to identify the type of pathologic motor response represented in the three patients illustrated below:

Decorticate
Decerebrate

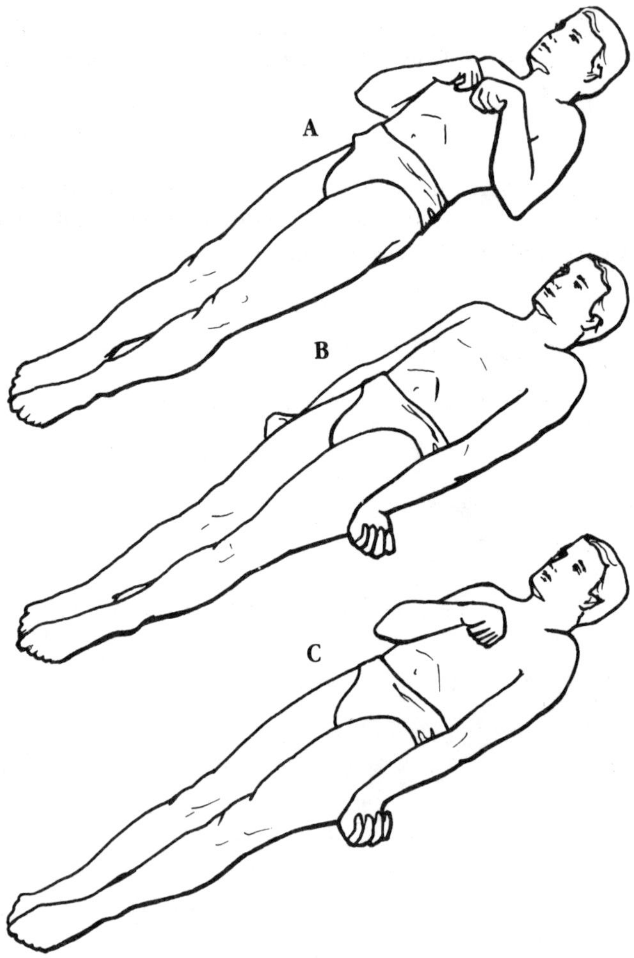

XVII. Circle the word that best describes each situation below.

May Zimmer, age 28, is in the intensive care unit because of multiple injuries she sustained in an automobile accident. She has been in the ICU for 5 days. Both legs are in traction and she is on bedrest. She is complaining of insomnia because of noise in the environment and being frequently awakened to have her vital signs checked. She is irritable and her appetite is diminishing.

1. On her eighth hospital day, she is unable to recall the year and her name. When asked if she knows where she is, she replies, "On my back porch in the swing."

   Confusion　　　Disorientation　　　Delirium

2. May becomes increasingly agitated each day. While the nurse is giving her hygienic care, May points to her IV bottle and IV pole and asks, "Who's that man? What's he going to do to us now?"

   Confusion　　　Illusion　　　Hallucination

3. On the tenth hospital day, the nurse observes May continually brushing her arms and the top bed cover. When asked what the problem is, May replies, "I'm trying to get rid of these tiny roaches crawling all over the place." The nurse looks and sees nothing crawling.

Disorientation Delirium Hallucination

4. Michael Cheney, age 26, has been unresponsive to verbal and painful stimuli for 2 years. However, occasionally his eyes open and wander from side to side, but without awareness or response to his environment.

Vegetative state Locked-in state Obtunded

5. Melinda Links, age 54, was in an automobile accident and suffered a severe head injury. She makes no response to verbal stimuli and responds only to painful stimuli by withdrawing her arm and frowning her face when pressure is applied to the nailbeds of her hand.

Vegetative state Locked-in state Light coma

XVIII. Multiple choice

Bobby Holter, age 20, has been diagnosed with migraine headaches.

1. Which of the following medications would most likely be prescribed as treatment for Bobby's headache?
   a. Aspirin
   b. Ergotamine tartrate
   c. Amitriptyline (Elavil)
   d. Advil
2. The nurse should understand that to help Bobby control his headaches, he must first:
   a. Recognize the types
   b. Determine its frequency
   c. Recognize its characteristics
   d. Identify its source
3. On assessment of Bobby, which of the following findings would be most characteristic of migraine headaches?
   a. Prodromal symptoms before the attack
   b. Tearing of the eyes
   c. Sustained contraction of neck muscles
   d. Sweating
4. When a person experiences loss or decreased sensation of pain, temperature, touch, and proprioception, either singularly or in combination, the major nursing concern will be meeting their need for:
   a. Communication
   b. Elimination
   c. Nutrition
   d. Safety
5. Rehabilitation of the person experiencing alterations in sensory and perceptual function focuses on:
   a. Teaching the patient and the family how to adapt by using unaffected senses
   b. Helping the patient locate miracle workers
   c. Helping the patient and family focus on the person's loss of function
   d. Helping the family learn how to do everything for the patient to reduce the patient's sense of loss
6. When caring for a patient with aphasia, you should:
   a. Talk loudly so he or she can hear you
   b. Refrain from giving explanations about procedures because they cannot understand them anyway
   c. Provide as much environmental stimuli as possible to prevent feelings of isolation
   d. Consider the type that the person has and adapt communications methods accordingly

7. When a lesion involves the lower motor neurons, the outcome seen may be all of the following *except:*
   a. Flaccid muscles
   b. Muscle rigidity
   c. Loss of reflexes
   d. Atrophy of the involved muscle
8. The prominent findings in individuals who have lesions of the extrapyramidal tract include all *except:*
   a. Muscle rigidity
   b. Bradykinesia without loss of strength
   c. Gross spasticity with voluntary movements
   d. Involuntary rest tremors that decrease when limb is used
9. Where do the majority of the upper motor neurons cross over (decussate) before they descend in the spinal cord?
   a. Cerebrum
   b. Pons
   c. Medulla
   d. Precentral gyrus
10. If a patient experiences an upper motor neuron lesion above the medulla in the left hemisphere of the cerebrum, you would expect the patient to have:
    a. Left-sided paresis or hemiplegia
    b. Right-sided paresis or hemiplegia
    c. Paralysis or weakness of both lower legs
    d. Paralysis or weakness of all extremities
11. All of the following interventions are aimed at preventing deformity in the patient with complete loss of motor function *except:*
    a. Positioning in good body alignment
    b. Providing range-of-motion exercises regularly
    c. Keeping the person in a semi-Fowler's position
    d. Using counterpositioning
12. A patient has a proprioception deficit. This means that the patient:
    a. Has numbness in the extremities
    b. Cannot recognize the position of his or her body and its parts with eyes closed
    c. Lacks the ability to control body temperature
    d. Loses balance when standing with eyes closed
13. Lower motor neurons consist of:
    a. Anterior horn cells located in the anterior gray matter of the spinal cord
    b. Posterior horn cells located in the posterior gray matter of the spinal cord
    c. Peripheral nerve fibers only
14. Muscle weakness occurs with both upper and lower motor neuron lesions. Which of the following factors would provide the best clue as to whether muscle weakness is due to an upper motor neuron lesion or a lower motor neuron lesion?
    a. Duration of weakness
    b. Onset of weakness
    c. Distribution of weakness
    d. Degree of weakness
15. Findings that are most characteristic of an upper motor neuron lesion include all *except:*
    a. Spasticity
    b. Clonus
    c. Hyperreflexia
    d. Muscle fasciculations
16. A person who has an upper motor neuron lesion below the medulla on the left side of the spinal cord will most likely experience:
    a. Left-sided alterations in motor function
    b. Right-sided alterations in motor function
    c. Alterations in motor function in all extremities
    d. None of the above

17. Which foods would *not* be contraindicated for persons with migraine headaches?
    a. Chocolate
    b. Nuts
    c. Caffeinated coffee
    d. Onions
18. The underlying pathophysiology of vascular headache is:
    a. Constriction of cerebral blood vessels
    b. Dilation of cerebral blood vessels
    c. Obstruction of cerebral blood vessels
    d. Hypoxia of cerebral tissue
19. Which statement about cluster headaches is incorrect?
    a. They start and stop abruptly.
    b. The onset is preceded by an aura.
    c. They may recur several times a day over several days.
    d. They are usually unilateral.
20. Tension headaches:
    a. Are related to fatique and stress
    b. Usually start in the infraorbital region
    c. Are primarily caused by hypertension
    d. Are characterized by nasal congestion and tearing
21. The major complication associated with untreated increased ICP is:
    a. Hypertension
    b. Renal failure
    c. Blindness
    d. Brain herniation
22. Care of the person experiencing a headache would include all *except:*
    a. Applying warm, dry compresses to the forehead and neck
    b. Teaching relaxation techniques
    c. Applying pressure to the temporal artery
    d. Providing a quiet, dark environment
23. Which of the following questions is *least* important when assessing a person experiencing a headache?
    a. Is the person taking oral contraceptives?
    b. Is there a family history of migraines?
    c. What is the person's age?
    d. Is the person fasting?
24. The earliest manifestation of increasing ICP is?
    a. Rising blood pressure
    b. Decreasing level of consciousness
    c. Decreasing pulse rate
    d. Change in the size of pupils
25. Which position would be best for the patient who is either experiencing or is high-risk for increasing ICP.
    a. Semi-Fowler's
    b. Flat, supine
    c. Flat, prone
    d. Any position of comfort

XIX. Write answers in the space provided.

1. List four guidelines for providing care to the patient experiencing root pain.

2. List six factors that can activate pain receptors.

3. List five causes of increasing ICP.

4. List three drugs that can be used to control spasticity in patients with neuromuscular disease.

5. List four conditions that are associated with alterations in movement and posture.

6. List five causes of headaches.

XX. Complete the chart on trigeminal neuralgia.

	Trigeminal neuralgia
Sex most prevalent in	
Cause	
Cranial nerve involved	
Clinical manifestations	
Activities to prevent pain	
Drugs used in its treatment	
Major problem to assess for if upper branch of nerve cut during surgery	
Major problem to assess for if lower branch of nerve cut during surgery	

XXI. Select the best answer for each item.

Mrs. Baker, age 41, is admitted to the hospital with a diagnosis of Guillain-Barré syndrome.

1. On assessment of Mrs. Baker, the nurse would anticipate finding all *except:*
a. Progressive motor weakness beginning with the lower extremities and progressing upward
b. Muscle tenderness and nerve sensitivity to pressure
c. An extremely elevated temperature
d. A history of exposure to a viral infection

2. Mrs. Baker is very depressed and says to the nurse, "I'll never be able to walk again. I might as well be dead." The nurse should base her response on a knowledge that:
a. Patients with Guillain-Barré can have a complete recovery without residual effects
b. Guillain-Barré is a progressive disorder that is manifested by periods of remission and exacerbations
c. Guillain-Barré can effectively be controlled with the use of anticholinergic drugs
d. Care for the patient is focused on helping the patient prepare for dying

An elderly male is brought to the emergency room by his wife because of generalized weakness, difficulty swallowing, chewing, and speaking. The patient's medical record indicates a history of myasthenia gravis. The doctor suspects that the patient is in myasthenia crisis and plans a edrophonium (Tensilon) test.

3. Which of the following drugs should the nurse have available when the Tensilon test is performed?
a. Prostigmine
b. Sinemet
c. Atropine Sulfate
d. L-dopa

4. The patient would be in myasthenia crisis if:
a. He showed a rapid improvement when Tensilon is given
b. His condition worsened when Tensilon was administered
c. His condition remained unchanged when Tensilon was administered

5. A patient with Parkinson's disease is admitted to the hospital. On assessment of the patient, you would expect to find all of the following *except:*
a. Rigidity, especially on passive movement of limbs
b. Pin-rolling tremors that are maximal at rest
c. Decreased motor power
d. Altered intellectual abilities

6. The most prominent manifestation of myasthenia gravis is:
a. Profound muscle weakness
b. Ataxic gait
c. Pin-rolling tremors
d. Spastic paralysis

7. Which of the following drugs is used in the primary treatment of petit mal seizures?
a. Mysoline
b. Dilantin
c. Zarontin
d. Tegretol

Karen Jacobs, age 21, is admitted to your clinical unit with a diagnosis of meningitis.

8. On assessment of Karen you would expect to find a history of:
a. Gastritis
b. Urinary tract infection
c. Hypertension
d. Respiratory tract infection

9. Nursing care of Karen would include all of the following *except:*
a. Respiratory isolation
b. Administration of antibiotics
c. Providing increased environmental stimulation
d. Providing adequate hydration

Becky Marino, age 19, fell off a log while at camp and hit her head on the ground. Reportedly Becky experienced temporary loss of consciousness at the time of the fall. Skull x-ray examination showed no cerebral damage.

10. Which type of head injury has Becky experienced?
  a. Concussion
  b. Contusion

11. Becky is discharged home. Becky's parents should be instructed to do all of the following *except:*
  a. Awaken her every hour when she is asleep for the first 24 hours
  b. Notify the physician immediately if she complains of a mild headache
  c. Contact the physician if she experiences double vision, forceful vomiting, or unusual sleepiness
  d. Have her sleep with one to two pillows

12. Six months later, Becky is brought to the emergency room. She was hit by a car while riding her bicycle. She has a severe head injury and is presently unconscious. Which nursing goal would be top priority at this time?
  a. Providing adequate nutrition
  b. Maintaining a patent airway
  c. Preventing fluid and electrolyte imbalance
  d. Preventing contractures

13. The nurse observes serosanguineous fluid oozing from Becky's left ear. You check the drainage with Tes-Tape. It is positive for glucose. The nurse should:
  a. Place her on her right side
  b. Keep her flat in bed
  c. Check for a history of diabetes mellitus
  d. Cover her left ear with a sterile dressing

14. With a lower motor neuron impairment, what symptoms are present?
  a. Reflexes are intact
  b. Patient experiences urinary retention
  c. Bladder empties automatically without control
  d. Bladder is hypertonic

Mindy Barlow, age 18, was in an automobile accident and sustained complete transection of the spinal cord at the lumbosacral area. She has no voluntary movements of her legs and is experiencing spastic movement of the legs. Mindy asks how long it will be before she can walk again.

15. Your response should be based on a knowledge that:
  a. Once swelling of the spinal cord has subsided she will be able to walk again
  b. Permanent flaccid paralysis will follow spastic movements
  c. Autoregeneration of the spinal cord takes about 1 to 2 years
  d. Rigorous physical therapy will be required to help her regain use of her legs

16. Which of the following manifestations would indicate overdrainage of a ventricular shunt in a patient who has the shunt implanted because of hydrocephalus?
  a. Hypertension
  b. Nausea and vomiting
  c. Diplopia
  d. Headache

XXII. Complete the chart on the following drugs.

Drug	Classification/action	Adverse effects	Nursing considerations
Ergotamine tartrate			
Dexamethasone (Decadron)			

You suspect that your patient with a stroke has aphasia. You perform gross testing to determine the type of aphasia by laying the following objects on the overbed table in front of the patient: a key, a pencil, a safety pin, and a book.

Write what you would have the person do with the above objects to assess for each of the types of aphasia listed below.

Types of aphasia	Assessments
Sensory	
Motor	
Global	

CASE STUDY

Maude Paulson, a 58-year-old obese secretary, is brought to the emergency room by her husband. He reports that while they were eating dinner, his wife suddenly slumped over in the chair and became unresponsive. On examination of her you find that she has ptosis of the left eye and sagging of the facial muscles on the left side of her face. She is drooling saliva from the left side of her mouth. Her left cheek puffs out with each expiration. She blinks her eyes sluggishly and looks around but does not respond to verbal command. She moves her left arm and leg spontaneously, but movement is slow. She has no movement in the right arm and leg, which are flaccid. She is incontinent of urine. Vital signs are: 98.8° F, 88(regular), 26(even), 220/112.

Mr. Paulson states that his wife has been on high blood pressure medication for 2 years and that she had stopped taking it about 3 months ago because she said that her blood pressure problem had been cured.

The physician suspects a CVA and orders a CT scan. The results of the scan reveal cerebral thrombosis.

Mr. Paulson asks, "Will my wife remain in this state for the rest of her life?" He also adds, "A friend of ours had a stroke about 2 years ago and only lost his ability to talk clearly. Why is my wife's stroke much worse than his?"

1. What would be the most appropriate response to Mr. Paulson's first question about the outcome for his wife?
2. What would be the most appropriate response to Mr. Paulson's second question about the differences in manifestations of a stroke?
3. How does the onset of symptoms differ in stroke caused by thrombosis, embolism, and aneurysm?
4. In which hemisphere of the brain did cerebral thrombosis occur in Mrs. Paulson?
5. Complete the nursing care plan below on Mrs. Paulson. From the above case study, write additional assessment data in the assessment column and then follow through with each phase.
6. If Mrs. Paulson was in your community, what resources would be available to assist in her rehabilitation?

NURSING CARE PLAN

Assessment	Nursing diagnosis	Goals	Interventions	Evaluation
Ptosis of left lid with sluggish blink reflex			Monitor for dryness of cornea, may need artificial tears.	
Flaccid; paralysis of left arm and leg; sluggish; spontaneous movement of right arm and leg	Impaired physical mobility R/T: left-sided paralysis			

CLINICAL ACTIVITIES

Perform the following neurologic tests on a peer and chart your findings:

a. Peripheral vision
b. Visual acuity
c. Romberg test
d. Coordination of muscle movements
e. Pupillary responses
f. Muscle strength
g. Twelve cranial nerves

SUGGESTED READINGS

Anderson, MS: Assessment under pressure: when your patient says, "My head hurts," Nursing 14:34-41, Sept 1984.
Describes the neurologic assessment of a patient for ICP, and nursing interventions to prevent ICP. Provides a chart showing stages of neurologic dysfunction based on assessment findings.

Arrowsmith, FM: Tenacious headaches, RN 46:29-35, Oct 1983.
Provides a guide for assessment of the patient with a headache, and describes each type of headache in relation to epidemiology, causes, signs and symptoms, and treatments.

Bell, J, and Hannon, K: Pathophysiology involved in autonomic dysreflexia, J Neurosci Nurs 18:86-87, April 1986.
Defines the syndrome, causes, manifestations, and appropriate management.

Callahan, ME: Caring for a stroke patient—like me, Nursing 14:65-67, May 1984.
Excellent article. The author, a nurse who experienced a stroke, describes some helpful suggestions on caring for the CVA patient based upon personal experiences.

Ellis, K: What to say about sex, RN 49:54-55, June 1986.
Discusses how to determine the right patient and right time to discuss sexual concerns with the stroke patient, how to help the person adjust to motor deficits and incontinence.

Gary, R, and others: Stroke: how to contain the damage, RN 49:36-41, May 1986.

Kess, R: Suddenly a crisis—unpredictable myasthenia, Am J Nurs 84:994-998, Aug 1984.

Chapter 20

The Patient with Eye Problems

CAROLE A. KAUFMANN

CHAPTER OBJECTIVES

On completion of this chapter, the student should be able to:

- Describe measurement and alterations in visual acuity and types of corrective lenses.
- Identify eye safety measures.
- Identify nursing interventions for the newly blind person.
- Describe major eye inflammations and appropriate nursing interventions.
- Explain the nature of cataracts, glaucoma, and retinal detachment and appropriate interventions.
- Describe the care of the person having eye surgery.

PREREQUISITE READING

Long-Phipps, Chapter 20, pp. 515-545.

SELF-ASSESSMENT ACTIVITIES

I. Define the following terms.

Accommodation
Block E chart
Cataract
Conjunctivitis
Dermatochalasis
Enophthalmos
Entropion
Exophthalmos
Hyperopia
Keratoplasty
Myopia
OD
OS
OU
Snellen chart
Styes
Trabeculum

II. Identify external eye structures on the illustration below.

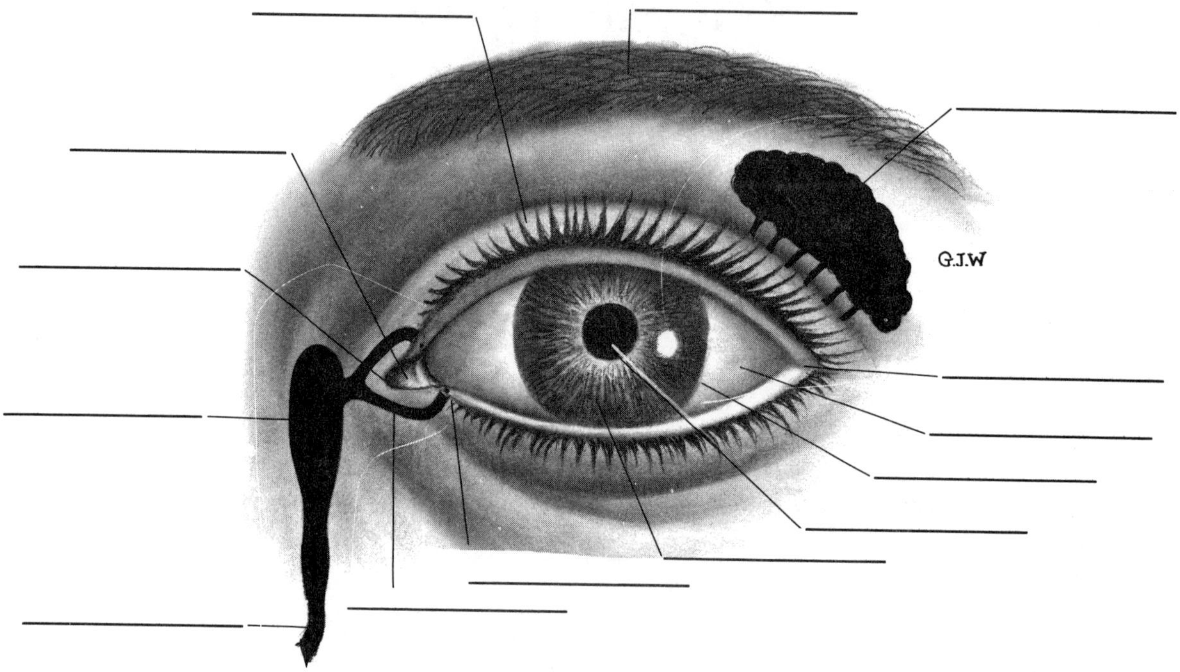

III. Identify parts of the eye on the illustration below of a horizontal section through left eyeball.

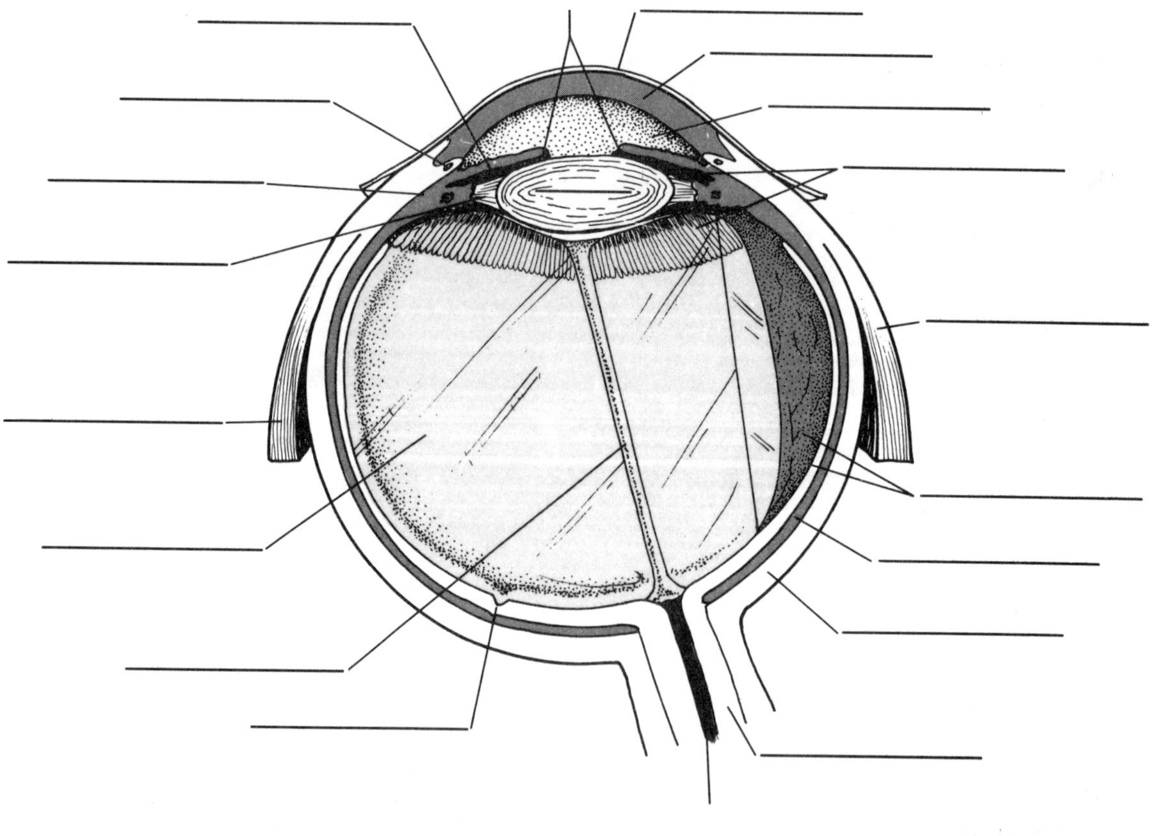

IV. Compare the soft contact lens with the hard contact lens in terms of advantages and disadvantages.

	Soft contact lens	Hard contact lens
Advantages		
Disadvantages		

V. Write answers to each of the following questions in the space provided.

1. When should persons of each of the following age groups have an eye examination?
 a. Children and young adults

 b. Middle-aged and older adults

2. How is a contact lens held in place?

3. What is the average healing time for a corneal graft? Why?

4. Describe the nursing goals of postoperative care following cataract surgery.

5. Which technique of cataract extraction involves removal of the anterior portion of the capsule plus the capsule content?

6. When the lens has been removed with cataract surgery, what three means are available for restoring focusing power in the operative eye?

7. When are cataract glasses generally prescribed?

8. What is the normal range of intraocular pressure?

9. What are the three most frequent causes of detached retina?

10. Why is atropine sulfate contraindicated for the patient with narrow-angle glaucoma?

11. What are the two legal criteria of blindness?

12. List four activities that patients should avoid after eye surgery because they can cause increased intraocular pressure.

VI. Match the terms with the approriate definition below.

a. Rhodopsin
b. Canal of Schlemm
c. Snellen chart
d. Refractive error
e. Palpebrae
f. Presbyopia
g. Astigmatism
h. Conjunctiva
i. Optician
j. Tonometer

1. _____ Person who grinds and fits lenses
2. _____ Visual disturbance caused by the image not being clearly focused on the retina
3. _____ Visual disturbance caused by abnormal curvature of the cornea
4. _____ Device used to measure ocular tension
5. _____ Card for assessing vision
6. _____ Tubular chamber that provides a pathway for aqueous humor to exit the eye
7. _____ Eyelids
8. _____ Transparent mucous membrane that covers the inner surface of the eyelids
9. _____ Blurring of near objects associated with the aging process
10. _____ A photosensitive protein essential for night vision

VII. Write the answers to the following questions in the space provided.

1. What is the relationship between vitamin A, rhodopsin, and night vision?

2. How is the lens held in place?

3. What is the normal distance vision?

4. Based upon results of a vision screening using a Snellen chart, when should a person be referred to an ophthalmologist?

5. When a person is given an appointment for an eye examination in which a cycloplegic drug will be used, what should the patient be told?

6. What is the pathway by which aqueous humor exits the eye?

VIII. Multiple choice

1. The receptors in the eye for bright daylight and color vision are:
a. Rods
b. Cones
c. Lens
d. Cornea

2. The receptors in the eye for dim or night vision are:
a. Rods
b. Cones
c. Lens
d. Cornea

3. Which statement about aqueous humor is *incorrect?*
   a. It is produced in the cornea.
   b. It is a clear liquid.
   c. It passes through the pupil into the anterior chamber.
   d. It exits the eye by way of the canal of Schlemm.
4. Which of the following does *not* occur when the eye accommodates to near vision?
   a. The ciliary body contracts.
   b. The suspensory ligament attached to the lens relaxes.
   c. The lens thickens.
   d. The pupil dilates.
5. Which of the following findings would not be considered a normal process of aging?
   a. Arcus senilis
   b. Presbyopia
   c. Senile miosis
   d. Ptosis
6. To assess ocular tension, the examiner will use a(an):
   a. Tonometer
   b. Ophthalmoscope
   c. Snellen chart
   d. Jaeger chart
7. With the person looking straight ahead at a target, you shine a penlight on the cornea to assess ocular movements. Your findings are normal. To record your findings you would write:
   a. There is consensual pupil constriction.
   b. There is no photosensitivity.
   c. The corneal reflex is in the same position on each pupil.
   d. Does not blink excessively when light is shined on the eye.
8. A person's distance vision is 20/40. This means that:
   a. The person was standing 40 feet from the chart and could only see at a distance of 20 feet
   b. The person can see at 20 feet what a person with normal vision can see at 40 feet
   c. The person can see at 40 feet what a normal person could see at 20 feet
   d. The person is legally blind
9. A school nurse is scheduled to perform visual acuity testing a group of 2-year-olds. The nurse should do all of the following *except:*
   a. Have the child stand 20 feet from the chart
   b. Use a chart with large numbers
   c. Record findings as a fraction
   d. Test each eye separately
10. Which statement regarding the posterior chamber of the eye is *incorrect?*
    a. It is the largest cavity of the eye.
    b. It contains a clear gel-like substance.
    c. It contains vitreous humor.
    d. It functions as a reservoir for excess aqueous humor.

Mrs. Barren, age 45, has returned to your clinical unit following a left keratoplasty. She has a metal eye shield over the left eye.

11. Three days following the corneal graft, Mrs. Barren states, "My vision is worse now than it was before the operation. Something must be wrong." Your response to the patient would be based upon an understanding that:
    a. Vision will improve once the sutures have been removed
    b. Diminished vision after surgery is an indication that the operation was not successful
    c. The patient needs to have a steroid eye drop to reduce swelling
    d. Glasses will be needed in order to improve the patient's vision

12. Which of the following discharge instructions would not be appropriate for Mrs. Barren?
    a. Check for graft rejection daily for the rest of your life.
    b. Report eye problems that persist or increase in severity in a 24-hour period.
    c. Check your eye at the same time each day.
    d. Return to the doctor's office within a week after discharge from the hospital for removal of the sutures.
13. Mrs. Barren should be told that all of the following are manifestations of a corneal graft rejection *except:*
    a. Redness
    b. Irritation
    c. Decrease in vision
    d. Severe eye pain
14. The most common cause of cataracts is:
    a. Trauma
    b. Aging
    c. Congenital defects
    d. Infections
15. The primary manifestation of cataracts is:
    a. Eye pain
    b. Progressive loss of vision
    c. Redness and swelling of the eye
    d. Night blindness
16. A patient has had bilateral cataract extraction. Cataract glasses have been prescribed for the patient. Which statement about cataract glasses would be inappropriate?
    a. The glasses will make everything appear closer.
    b. Clear vision is possible only through the center of the lens of the glasses.
    c. The glasses will restore sight with extended use.
    d. Colors seen from the operated eye are slightly distorted.
17. Which pathophysiological finding does not occur in glaucoma?
    a. Increased intraocular pressure
    b. Decrease in the amount of vitreous humor
    c. Loss of peripheral vision
    d. Increase in the amount of aqueous humor
18. Which of the following instructions would be appropriate for the patient with glaucoma?
    a. Eye medications will have to be used for the rest of your life.
    b. Vision loss can be restored with continued use of eye medications.
    c. Reduce fluid intake to control intraocular pressure.
    d. Avoid excess use of your eyes.
19. Preoperative care of the patient with a detached retina of the left eye in the temporal region would include all *except:*
    a. Covering both eyes
    b. Keeping the patient in a left lateral position
    c. Allowing the patient to ambulate in his room only
    d. Administering mydriatic eye drops
20. Which of the following surgical procedures is used for retinal detachment?
    a. Iridectomy
    b. Trabeculectomy
    c. Keratoplasty
    d. Scleral buckling
21. Which type of drugs should not be given to a patient with a detached retina?
    a. Mydriatics
    b. Cycloplegics
    c. Steroids
    d. Miotics

22. When caring for a patient with visual impairment or who is blind, you should:
    a. Talk loudly so the patient can understand you
    b. Avoid use of such phrases as "See what I mean"
    c. Introduce yourself with each contact
    d. Refrain from spending too much time with the patient
23. Mrs. Lentz, age 60, is scheduled for an extracapsular cataract extraction. Preoperatively, she will most likely receive any of the following drugs *except:*
    a. Mydriatics
    b. Miotics
    c. Osmotic agents
    d. Cycloplegics
24. Mrs. Lentz returns to your clinical unit after surgery. She has a metal eyeshield over the left eye. Nursing care for her would include:
    a. Position her on the unaffected side
    b. Remove the eye shield when she is safely in bed
    c. Position her on the affected side
    d. Have patient shower
25. To keep healthy eyes healthy, individuals should be advised to:
    a. Cleanse the eyes daily with a solution such as Visine
    b. Cleanse the eyes daily with a solution of Boric acid
    c. Consume megadoses of vitamin A
    d. Look away at a distance periodically when doing extremely fine work at a very close distance
26. Your next-door neighbor is complaining of severe pain in the eye and blurred vision. This person should be referred to an:
    a. Optometrist
    b. Ophthalmologist
    c. Optician
27. To irrigate an individual's left eye, you should:
    a. Warm the irrigating solution to 100° F
    b. Direct a forceful stream of the solution onto the eye to ensure removal of debris
    c. Have patient hold emesis basin to cheek with head tilted to the left
    d. Direct the solution to flow from the outer canthus to inner canthus
28. When performing a thorough fundoscopic examination, which type of eye medication would the ophthalmologist most likely use?
    a. Miotics
    b. Mydriatics
    c. Osmotic agents
    d. Carbonic anhydrase inhibitors
29. Which type of drug would be contraindicated for the patient with glaucoma?
    a. Miotics
    b. Mydriatics
    c. Osmotic agents
    d. Carbonic anhydrase inhibitors
30. To prevent systemic absorption of ophthalmic solutions, you should:
    a. Give exactly what is ordered and no more
    b. Have the patient squeeze eyes tightly after instilling the eye drops
    c. Flush the eyes after instilling the eye drops
    d. Have patient tilt head forward
31. The primary reason that an eye ointment would be prescribed over eye drops is that:
    a. Ointments remain in contact with the eye much longer than eye drops
    b. Ointments are not as messy as eye drops
    c. Ointment seldom interfere with vision
    d. Ointments are absorbed into the lacrimal duct much faster than are eye drops

32. Nutritional deficiencies commonly cause pathologic changes in all of the following components of the eye *except:*
    - **a.** Retina
    - **b.** Cornea
    - **c.** Conjunctiva
    - **d.** Blood vessels
33. While on a hike through the woods, your partner is hit in the eye with a tree branch. He is moaning loudly and holding his hand over his left eye. You manage to pry his hand away and observe a small piece of tree bark protruding from his eyelid. Before transporting him to the nearest medical facility, you should:
    - **a.** Remove the piece of tree bark from his eyelid
    - **b.** Flush both eyes with water
    - **c.** Cover both eyes
    - **d.** Apply an ice compress to the left eye
34. Which statement about acute bacterial conjunctivitis is correct?
    - **a.** It can be transmitted by direct contact.
    - **b.** It always leaves permanent scarring of the cornea.
    - **c.** It is highly contagious.
    - **d.** It is self-limiting and requires no treatment.
35. Which of the following eye disorders leads to blindness?
    - **a.** Trachoma
    - **b.** Conjunctivitis
    - **c.** Chalazion
    - **d.** Styes

IX. For each of the eye problems listed below, write in the space provided the treatments for each.

Problem	Treatment
Lacerations of eyelid	
Ecchymosis	
Chalazion	
Conjunctivitis	
Chemical injuries to eye	
Dirt or debris in eyes	
Uveitis	
Styes	
Keratitis	

X. Compare the two types of intraocular lens implants listed by completing the information in the chart below.

	Anterior chamber lens	Posterior chamber lens
Where is the lens placed?		
What type of cataract extraction procedure is used?		
What supports the lens once it is in place?		
Which type is most popular and why?		

XI. Match the type of glaucoma described by each of the statements below.

a. Open-angle (chronic, simple)
b. Angle-closure (narrow angle)

1. _____ Caused by obstruction in the trabecular meshwork
2. _____ Surgical treatment includes an iridectomy
3. _____ Characterized by acute severe eye pain with decreased vision
4. _____ Surgical treatment involves a trabeculectomy
5. _____ Characterized by progressive loss of peripheral vision
6. _____ Eyes are red with steamy cornea and fixed, dilated pupil
7. _____ Closing of the angle between the iris and cornea
8. _____ Characterized by persistent, dull eye pain

XII. Compare the two types of intraocular lens implants listed by completing the information in the chart below.

Type	Action	Clinical uses	Name of agent commonly used
Mydriatics			
Miotics			
Osmotic agents			
Carbonic anhydrase inhibitors			
Cycloplegics			

CLINICAL ACTIVITIES

1. Cover both eyes at home for 1 hour and attempt to carry on your daily routine. What problems did you encounter? What were your greatest fears?
2. Cover one eye at home for 1 hour and attempt to carry on your daily routine. What problems did you encounter? What adjustment did you have to make?
3. What services are available in your community to assist the blind or visually impaired?
4. Have you ever interacted with or taken care of a blind person? What were your initial thoughts about the person? What adjustments did you make to allow or encourage the person to maintain independence?

SUGGESTED READINGS

Alven, MT: Ophthalmic prosthetics: a guide for nurses (pictorial), 6:218-223, Nov/Dec 1987.

Capeno, DG, and others: Age-related macular degeneration (pictorial), Hos Pract 23(3);23-25, 29-30, 36-38, 1988.

Hahn, AB, and others: Overview of the eye and ophthalmic agents, In Mosby's pharmacology in nursing, St Louis, 1986, The CV Mosby Co.

Hunt, L: Use of the Honon intraocular pressure reducer (pictorial), J Ophthalmic Nurs Technol 7(2):59-61, 1988.

Manser, JH, and others: Intraocular inflammatory disease (uveitis), Ophthalmic Nurs Forum 4(1):1-8, 1988.

Chapter 21

The Patient with Ear Problems

BRENDA GOODNER

CHAPTER OBJECTIVES

On completion of this chapter, the student should be able to:

- Describe the mechanics of sound waves and hearing.
- Describe measures to prevent hearing loss.
- Describe the pathophysiology and nursing requirements for persons with ear infections.
- Describe the pathophysiology and care of the person with a balance disorder.
- Describe care of the person having ear surgery.
- Differentiate conductive and sensorineural hearing loss and describe methods of assessment.
- Describe methods of aural rehabilitation and communication with hearing impaired persons.

PREREQUISITE READING

Long-Phipps, Chapter 21, pp. 547-567.

SELF-ASSESSMENT ACTIVITIES

I. Define the following terms.

Audiometirc testing
Conductive hearing loss
Eardrum
Eustachian tube
External ear
Hearing threshold
Inner ear
Mastoid
Middle ear
Otitis
Otology
Otosclerosis
Otoscope
Sensorineural hearing loss
Tympanic membrane
Vertigo

II. Match the following characteristics of sound.

a. Sensation of sound intensity
b. Number of sound waves per second emanating from a source
c. Pressure exerted by a sound measured in decibels
d. Sensation of sound frequency experienced by a person

1. _____ Intensity
2. _____ Loudness
3. _____ Frequency
4. _____ Pitch

III. Answer the following questions.

1. What three classifications of drugs adversely affect hearing?

2. What are the two major symptoms of external and middle ear infections?

3. What solution is used for an ear wash?

4. What solution is used for an ear irrigation?

5. List seven nursing interventions for instillation of ear drops.

6. List five drugs that may be prescribed for a patient with vertigo.

IV. Multiple choice

1. Dizziness is a very common complaint and is often associated with inner ear problems. The medical term for dizziness is:
   a. Tinnitus
   b. Labyrinthitis
   c. Sensorineural
   d. Vertigo
2. The priority nursing responsibility in caring for a patient with dizziness is:
   a. Safety
   b. Comfort
   c. Hygiene
   d. Nausea
3. The major purpose of a hearing aid is to:
   a. Improve ability to hear
   b. Make sounds louder
   c. Pick up vocal sounds only
   d. Facilitate communication
4. The appropriate method of administering ear drops to an adult is:
   a. Pull the ear down and forward
   b. Pull the ear up and back
   c. Pull the ear down and back
   d. Stabilizing the ear in its normal position
5. The physician requests that the nurse assist with the insertion of ear wicks into a patient's ear canal. The nurse gathers the appropriate equipment, which includes:
   a. Mayo scissors
   b. Bandage scissors
   c. Alligator forceps
   d. Bayonet forceps
6. Mr. Simon, 48, has chronic ear infections and is instructed to wash his ears with an ear wash once a week. He is taught that the most commonly prescribed ear wash solution is:
   a. Plain water
   b. Normal saline
   c. Boric acid and alcohol
   d. Hydrogen peroxide and water
7. The first thing the nurse should check when a hearing aid is not working is:
   a. The battery
   b. The on-off switch
   c. The cord plug
   d. The position of the earmold

8. Care of the hearing aid includes which of the following actions?
   a. Clean earmold once a month
   b. Avoid soap
   c. Use pipe cleaner to clean cannula
   d. Protect transmitter under clothing
9. Which of the following approaches facilitates communication with the hearing impaired?
   a. Smile frequently
   b. Speak loudly
   c. Talk directly into "good" ear
   d. Do not overaccentuate words
10. A nursing action to help the person with vertigo includes which of the following activities?
    a. Avoid sudden movements
    b. Avoid noises
    c. Encourage fluid intake
    d. Suggest patient lie on affected side
11. Loss of hearing may manifest itself in which of the following behaviors?
    a. Withdraws
    b. Becomes aggressive
    c. Repeats self
    d. Speaks loudly
12. The inner ear is a complex system composed of two major structures. Which of the following structures connects the semicircular canals and the cochlea?
    a. Vestibule
    b. Bony labyrinth
    c. Membranous labyrinth
    d. Scala vestibuli
13. Which of the following structures is the end organ for hearing?
    a. Endolymph
    b. Scala tympani
    c. Vestibular membrane
    d. Organ of Corti
14. Nerve impulses are transmitted between the ear and the brain by:
    a. Seventh cranial nerve
    b. Sixth cranial nerve
    c. Eighth cranial nerve
    d. Glossopharyngeal nerve
15. Sound is transmitted from the external ear to the inner ear by:
    a. Air and bone conduction
    b. Air and nerve conduction
    c. Air, bone and nerve conduction
    d. Bone and nerve conduction
16. The tympanic membrane is a thin, oval transparent membrane that:
    a. Is normally pink in color and retracted
    b. Is normally pearly gray in color
    c. Is normally white in color with a red border
    d. Is normally partly open to transmit sound

V. Write a teaching plan for the following.

1. A patient with an ear infection.

2. A patient who has just had ear surgery.

VI. Discuss ways to facilitate communication with a person who has impaired hearing.

SUGGESTED READING

Shea, JJ, and Archik, J: Archives of otolaryngology (research article—diagnostic assessment), 112:929-934, No 9, Sept 1986. Electrocochleography and low frequency harmonic acceleration in Meniere's disease. Clinical research of 31 cases of Meniere's disease using two electrophysiologic procedures, electrocochleography and low-frequency harmonic acceleration (HA). Table for criteria for selection of patients presenting with Meniere's disease. Tests for hearing loss and vertigo.

Chapter 22

The Patient with Musculoskeletal Disorders

JACQUELINE S. SPRAGUE

CHAPTER OBJECTIVES

On completion of this chapter, the student should be able to:

- Describe measures to prevent musculoskeletal dysfunction.
- Describe conservative health measures for persons with joint and muscle disorders.
- Describe the pathophysiologic changes and therapy for rheumatoid arthritis, SLE, degenerative joint disorders, and scoliosis.
- Explain the nature of and describe the care of the patient undergoing total hip and total knee replacement
- Describe the care of the patient undergoing spinal fusion.
- Identify different types of fractures and their treatment.
- Explain the pathophysiology of bone healing.
- Describe problems that may occur with immobilization.
- Describe care of the patient following closed and open reduction of hip fractures (including cast care and traction).

PREREQUISITE READING

Long-Phipps, Chapter 22, pp. 569-634.

SELF-ASSESSMENT ACTIVITIES

I. Define the following terms.

Arthrodesis
Arthroplasty
Balanced suspension traction
Bouchard's nodes
Buck's extension
Butterfly rash
Comminuted fracture
Crepitus
Diarthroses
Dupuytren's contracture
Extracapsular fracture
Heberden's nodes
Herniated nucleus pulposus
Internal fixation devices
Intracapsular fracture
Logrolling
Osteoarthritis
Osteophyte
Pannus
Petechiae
Rheumatoid factor
Russell traction
Synarthroses
Tophi
Ulnar deviation

II. Write your answers in the space provided.

1. List five measures that may be used to prevent musculoskeletal complications.

2. Compare the effects of heat and cold when used therapeutically in musculoskeletal dysfunction.

3. List guidelines for moving patients with musculoskeletal problems.

4. Name at least four assistive devices used for patients with musculoskeletal problems.

III. Completion

1. Using the format below, compare the inflammatory disorder *rheumatoid arthritis* with the degenerative joint disorder *osteoarthritis.*

Disorder	Etiology	Clinical presentation	Medical management and/or surgical management	Nursing management
Rheumatoid arthritis				
Osteoarthritis				

2. Discuss reconstructive surgery of the hip and knee, describing preoperative care, surgery, postoperative care, and discharge instructions.

Surgery	Preoperative care	Surgery	Postoperative care	Discharge instructions
Total hip replacement				
Total knee replacement				

3. Compare the pathophysiology, treatment, and nursing care of patients with carpal tunnel syndrome and Dupuytren's contracture.

Disorder	Pathophysiology	Clinical presentation	Medical management
Carpal tunnel syndrome			
Dupuytren's contracture			

4. Describe the pathaphysiology, clinical presentation, and medical management of a patient with degenerative joint disease of the spine.

Degenerative disease of the spine	Pathophysiology	Clinical presentation	Medical management

5. Your patient, Mrs. Vale, is admitted to the orthopedic floor for a laminectomy with a spinal fusion. Write a nursing care plan for Mrs. Vale.

Assessment data	Nursing diagnosis	Outcomes	Interventions	Evaluation

6. Using the table below, list the characteristics, management, and examples of skin and skeletal traction.

Types	Characteristics	Management	Examples
Skin			
Skeletal			

IV. Matching

a. Break across bone
b. One bone fragment forcibly driven into another bone fragment
c. Bone broken, skin intact
d. Fracture parts extend through skin
e. Bone broken into several fragments
f. Splintering one side of bone only—bent

1. _____ Simple fracture
2. _____ Greenstick fracture
3. _____ Comminuted fracture
4. _____ Transverse fracture
5. _____ Compound fracture
6. _____ Impacted fracture

V. Multiple choice

Mr. Rombali, a 40-year-old fishing captain, is on the orthopedic unit with an acute exacerbation of rheumatoid arthritis.

1. Mr. Rombali's most urgent need is most likely to be:
   a. Relief from joint stiffness
   b. Interventions to increase activity
   c. Relief of pain
   d. Assistance with personal hygiene
2. Rheumatoid arthritis is generally classified as:
   a. An inflammatory disorder
   b. A disease of immune mechanism
   c. A genetic disorder
   d. A degenerative process
3. Systemic manifestations of rheumatoid arthritis include:
   a. Pain, redness of joints, subcutaneous nodules
   b. Excessive warmth in joints
   c. Hip joint tenderness
   d. Fever, weight loss, and fatigue
4. Which of Mr. Rombali's joints were probably affected early in his disease process?
   a. Patellar and ankle joints
   b. Ulnar and shoulder joints
   c. Metacarpophalangeal and proximal interphalangeal joints
5. A major factor in the management of Mr. Rombali's care is:
   a. Complete bed rest during the acute period of his disease
   b. Encouraging him to be as active as possible
   c. Ice packs to his affected joints
   d. Encouraging him to eat a high-caloric, low-salt diet
6. A potentially dangerous side effect of the nonsteroidal antiinflammatory drug naproxen (Naprosyn) is that it:
   a. Is irritating to the gastrointestinal tract
   b. Causes tinnitus and fluid retention
   c. Should not be taken with food
   d. Causes drowsiness
7. Mr. Rombali's rheumatologist prescribed the antiinflammatory drug prednisone 4 times a day. The nurse should know the side effects and precautions so that she can instruct Mr. Rombali and his wife. One of the major precautions when taking this drug on a once-a-day basis is:
   a. Take the dose in the morning
   b. Use for only 7 to 10 days
   c. Have an eye examination before starting drug
   d. Do not use when driving

8. Gold salt is also used in the medical management of rheumatoid arthritis. This drug causes which of the following major side effects?
   a. Lupuslike symptoms
   b. Retarded wound healing
   c. Hematologic changes
   d. Fever

Mr. Rombali was discharged after his acute exacerbation of the disease abated. However, the pain in his right hip became progressively worse and after 6 months, his doctor advised a total right hip replacement. He was admitted for a hip arthoplasty.

9. What type of preoperative teaching should be done to prepare Mr. Rombali for his postoperative period?
   a. Teach full range-of-motion (ROM) exercises for the right hip, because they will be started on his first postoperative day.
   b. Teach Mr. Rombali to keep his right leg in adduction at all times.
   c. Teach him how to turn from his back to the operative side after surgery.
10. Discharge instructions for Mr. Rombali include all of the following *except:*
   a. Limit right hip flexion to 90 degrees for about 2 months
   b. Avoid adduction of the right hip
   c. Make patient aware of lifelong need for prophylactic antibiotic therapy
   d. May put full weight-bearing on right leg without need of assistive devices after 1 week
11. Activity for a postoperative total knee replacement begins:
   a. On the fourth postoperative day with passive ROM to knee
   b. Immediately after surgery with the use of a continuous passive motion (CPM) machine
   c. Second day with straight leg raises
   d. After the drains are removed
12. Mrs. Onzoni has been admitted for surgery for right carpal tunnel syndrome. This means that:
   a. There is limited motion in the right elbow
   b. There is thickening of the palmar fascia of the right hand
   c. There is swelling over the dorsum of the right hand
   d. There is compression of the right medial nerve
13. The major postoperative intervention for Mrs. Onzoni would be:
   a. She may be up and about ad lib
   b. To check the neurocirculatory status of her right hand
   c. To keep her right arm down at her side
   d. To administer analgesics for pain
14. Gout is a metabolic disorder resulting from deposits of urate crystals in the synovial tissue resulting in pain, swelling, and erythema of the involved joints. Interventions for this disorder include all the following *except:*
   a. ROM to the point of resistance
   b. Absolute rest until the pain subsides
   c. Ensure good fluid intake
   d. Give medications as prescribed
15. Preventive therapy for gout includes the use of probenecid and allopurinal. Allopurinal works by which action?
   a. Enhancing uric acid excretion
   b. Promoting absorption of potassium in the tubules
   c. Lowering blood glucose levels
   d. Decreasing uric acid formation
16. One of the major points of information to teach a patient who has systemic lupus erythematosus is:
   a. To avoid returning to former job
   b. To be dependent
   c. How to avoid exposure to sunlight
   d. How to conceal facial lesions

Margie Tyson, age 67, slipped in her bathtub at home one evening while taking a shower. She was brought to the emergency room of the community hospital, where x-ray examination revealed an intertrochanteric fracture of the left hip. Margie was admitted to the orthopedic unit. Her left extremity was placed in 5 pounds Buck's traction. An overhead trapeze bar was placed on her bed.

17. On assessment of Margie, the nurse in the emergency room would expect to find all of the following *except*:
- **a.** Absence of a femoral pulse
- **b.** Loss of movement of the left leg
- **c.** Shortening and external rotation of the left leg
- **d.** Severe pain in the left hip area with movement

18. Nursing care for Margie while she is in Buck's traction would include:
- **a.** Ensuring that the weights rest securely on the floor
- **b.** Performing neurocirculatory checks
- **c.** Providing special care to the skin areas around the pin sites
- **d.** Removing the traction periodically to give skin care to the affected leg

19. Margie is taken to surgery and has an open reduction of her left hip with a nail insertion. Postoperative care for her would involve:
- **a.** Positioning her from side to side every 2 hours
- **b.** Maintaining the legs in adduction
- **c.** Assisting her to ambulate the first postoperative day with full weight-bearing
- **d.** Avoiding hip flexion beyond 60 degrees for 6 to 10 days

20. Which of the following preventive discharge instructions would be most appropriate for Margie?
- **a.** Advising her to use seat belts while driving
- **b.** Advising her to avoid drinking and driving
- **c.** Attaching safety arms around the toilet
- **d.** Having grab bars mounted on the wall next to the bathtub at home

Michael Muller, age 32, fell from a second story hotel balcony and sustained a partial fracture of the lumbar vertebrae. No other injuries were noted.

21. Nursing care for Michael includes:
- **a.** Logrolling him from side to side with a pillow between his legs every 2 hours
- **b.** Placing him in a Fowler's position to enhance breathing
- **c.** Applying a brace or corset after he gets out of bed
- **d.** Avoiding range-of-motion exercises to the lower extremities

22. The most important nursing assessments to make routinely of Michael include all the following *except:*
- **a.** Bowel and bladder elimination
- **b.** Sensation and movement in the lower extremities
- **c.** Circulation in the lower extremities
- **d.** Desire to learn a new skill

Omari Ingraham, age 8, fell off the swing at school. He is complaining of severe pain in his left lower arm. The school nurse is summoned.

23. To assess for the presence of a fracture of the patient's left arm the nurse should do all the following *except:*
- **a.** Move the arm in different positions to detect crepitus
- **b.** Look for obvious deformity
- **c.** Look for edema
- **d.** Look for inability to move his arm and fingers

24. The school nurse suspects a complete fracture of Omari's left lower arm. Immediate treatment would consist of all *except:*
- **a.** Splinting the arm to prevent movement
- **b.** Elevating the arm to reduce edema
- **c.** Applying heat to improve circulation
- **d.** Checking for adequate neurocirculation

Omari is taken to the emergency room of the community hospital, where x-ray examination reveals a complete fracture of the radius and partial fracture of the ulna. He is admitted to the hospital, and a closed reduction under general anesthesia is scheduled for the next day.

25. Nursing care for Omari during the initial 24 hours would include all *except:*
- **a.** Checking neurocirculation of his fingers every hour
- **b.** Using the palms of the hands to handle cast
- **c.** Elevating the arm on a pillow
- **d.** Applying heat to the casted arm

26. When Omari is ready for discharge, which of the following instructions would be inappropriate?
- **a.** Do not insert sharp objects in the cast
- **b.** Avoid getting the cast wet
- **c.** Keep arm elevated until swelling in fingers subsides
- **d.** To prevent soiling of the cast, paint over it with clear varnish

27. Traction may be used to accomplish all of the following *except:*
- **a.** Reduce a fracture
- **b.** Correct deformities
- **c.** Immobilize a limb
- **d.** Promote muscle contraction

Tom Jones, age 28, was in a motorcycle accident. X-ray examination admission revealed a comminuted fracture of his left femur and oblique fracture of his right tibia and fibula without displacement. His right leg was placed in a long leg cast and a pin was inserted through his left tibia, enabling his left leg to be placed in skeletal traction with balanced suspension.

28. The management of his traction will include all *except:*
- **a.** Keeping the weight steadied against the bedframe
- **b.** Leaving areas under knee and heel free from friction
- **c.** Encourage ROM to left ankle and foot
- **d.** Keeping all ropes running freely over the pulleys

29. A disadvantage of skeletal traction over skin traction is:
- **a.** Less freedom of movement in bed
- **b.** Skin traction can tolerate more weight
- **c.** Danger of infection
- **d.** Potential for nerve damage

Tom progressed well until 2 or 3 days after admission. When the nurse assisted Tom, she found him to be slightly confused and discovered petechiae on his chest and his conjunctiva.

30. She should immediately suspect which complication of fracture?
- **a.** Avascular necrosis
- **b.** Ischemic paralysis
- **c.** Osteomyelitis
- **d.** Fat embolism

SUGGESTED READINGS

Pryor, G, and others: Team management of the elderly patient with hip fracture, Lancet: 401 403, Feb 1988.
Kozinn, SC, and others: Adult hip disease and total hip replacement, Clin Symp 39(5):2-32, 1987.
Chamber, JK: Metabolic bone disorders: imbalances of calcium and phosphorus, Nurs Clin North Am (4):861-872, 1987.
Sabel, S: Osteoporosis: estrogen connection clearer, Am J Nurs Reg View Pub 1 Health Rep (1):13-14, 1988.

UNIT VI Gas Transport Problems

Chapter 23

The Patient with Nose and Throat Problems

BRENDA GOODNER

CHAPTER OBJECTIVES

On completion of this chapter, the student should be able to:

- Describe pathophysiologic bases of upper respiratory infections and therapeutic modalities.
- Describe nursing care of persons having nose and sinus surgery and tonsillectomy.
- Describe etiology and interventions for nosebleeds.
- Describe etiology and symptoms of cancer of the larynx and postoperative care following surgery.

PREREQUISITE READING

Long-Phipps, Chapter 23, pp. 637-663.

SELF-ASSESSMENT ACTIVITIES

I. Define the following terms.

Deviated septum
Esophageal speech
Laryngectomy
Laryngitis
Pharyngitis
Rhinitis
Rhinoplasty
Sinuses
Sinusitis
Tonsillitis
Turbinate bones

II. List the signs and symptoms of the following disorders.

Disorder	Signs and symptoms
Rhinitis (common cold)	
Allergic rhinitis (hay fever)	
Chronic rhinitis	
Acute sinusitis	
Chronic sinusitis	

III. Match the location of pain with sinusitis.

Pain location

a. Periorbital and frontal
b. Under eyes, front of face, dental, or eyes
c. Over eyebrow
d. Retroorbital, occipital, or top of head

Sinus

1. _____ Maxillary
2. _____ Frontal
3. _____ Ethmoid
4. _____ Sphenoid

IV. Multiple choice

1. Acute sinusitis must be treated with:
  a. Surgery
  b. Antibiotics
  c. Nasal sprays
  d. Aspirin

2. Why is a gross check of the patient's visual acuity important after sinus surgery?
  a. Orbital edema
  b. Damage to optic nerve
  c. Damage to trigeminal nerve
  d. Retinal detachment

3. Why is aspirin contraindicated after a tonsillectomy?
  a. Increases sensitization
  b. Increases bleeding tendency
  c. Irritation of pharynx
  d. Gastric irritation

4. What should the patient be told about probable throat discomfort after tonsillectomy?
  a. It will be minimal
  b. It will gradually become less
  c. It may be moderate for 3 days, then decrease
  d. It may increase slightly between fourth and eighth postoperative day

5. What is the most appropriate position for a patient when nose bleeding continues?
  a. Supine without a pillow
  b. Semi-Fowler's with head forward
  c. Supine with feet higher than head
  d. Side-lying with face toward mattress

6. It is important to check the position of a postnasal pack frequently because slippage can result in:
  a. Airway obstruction
  b. Severe apprehension
  c. Nausea and vomiting
  d. Increased restlessness

7. Which measure promotes comfort after nasal surgery?
  a. Suction the nose
  b. Apply an ice collar
  c. Provide mouth care
  d. Remove soiled nose splint

8. What is an early symptom of cancer of the larynx?
  a. Hoarseness
  b. Sore throat
  c. Neck swelling
  d. Enlarged lymph nodes of neck

9. What is the final effect on breathing following a total laryngectomy?
    a. Labored breathing through the mouth
    b. Labored breathing through nose
    c. Breathing through a temporary tracheostomy
    d. Breathing through a permanent tracheostomy
10. By what manner does a person talk after total laryngectomy?
    a. Normally
    b. Only through an electronic speech aid
    c. By esophageal speech
    d. By tracheal speech

Steve Wargo, age 50, experiences a nose bleed at home while sitting and watching television.

11. Most nose bleeds can be controlled by compressing the soft tissue of the nose against the septum for:
    a. 1 to 2 minutes
    b. 3 to 4 minutes
    c. 5 to 6 minutes
    d. 30 minutes or longer
12. To prevent recurrent epistaxis, Steve should be taught to:
    a. Eat foods high in vitamin K
    b. Breathe through the mouth
    c. Blow his nose gently
    d. Apply ice when nose feels irritated

V. Write a nursing care plan for the following.

1. The postoperative care of a patient undergoing sinus surgery.

2. The postoperative care of a patient undergoing nasal surgery.

VI. Answer the following questions in the space provided.

1. Why is aspirin not recommended for sinusitis?

2. What factors would be included in a patient teaching plan for a patient with sinusitis?

3. What are the common causes of nosebleeds?

VII. Discuss the correct administration of nose drops.

Chapter 24

The Patient with Pulmonary Problems

BRENDA GOODNER

CHAPTER OBJECTIVES

On completion of this chapter, the student should be able to:

- Differentiate between restrictive and obstructive pulmonary disorders.
- Describe the nature of viral respiratory infections and methods of assisting effective coughing.
- Compare classic, atypical, aspiration, and hematogenous pneumonia.
- Describe measures to promote oxygenation, facilitate breathing, and provide ventilation and hydration.
- Describe incidence, preventive measures, and therapeutic approaches to tuberculosis.
- Compare fungal infections of the respiratory tract.
- Explain the pathophysiology of adult respiratory distress syndrome (ARDS).
- Describe incidence, prevention, and therapy for lung cancer.
- Describe types of chest surgery and the care of the patient undergoing chest surgery (including patients with chest tubes).
- Describe the pathophysiologic conditions of chest trauma (for instance fractured ribs, penetrating wounds, and pneumothorax).
- Explain the pathophysiologic conditions and interventions for chronic obstructive pulmonary disease.
- Describe the nature of respiratory insufficiency and the care of the patient with an artificial airway or mechanical ventilation.

PREREQUISITE READING

Long-Phipps, Chapter 24, pp. 665-754.

SELF-ASSESSMENT

I. Define the following terms.

Adult respiratory distress syndrome (ARDS)
Arterial blood loss
Atelectasis
Aspiration pneumonia
Blastomycosis
Bronchitis
Bronchodilators
Bronchogenic carcinoma
Bronchoscopy
Cilia
Coccidioidomycosis
Diffusion
Dyspnea
Emphysema
Empyema
Expiratory reserve volume
Flail chest
Forced expiratory volume
Functional residual capacity
Goblet cells
Hemothorax
Histoplasmosis
Hyperventilation
Hypoventilation
Inspiratory capacity
Inspiratory reserve volume
Legionnaires' disease
Lobectomy
Lung compliance
Mantoux test
Maximal voluntary ventilation
Obstructive lung disease
Parietal pleura
Perfusion
Pleural effusion
Pneumoconioses
Pneumonectomy
Penumonia
Pneumothorax
Positive-end expiratory pressure (PEEP)
Potential space

Continued

Residual volume
Respiration
Thoracotomy
Tidal volume
Total lung capacity
Tuberculosis
Ventilation
Visceral pleura
Vital capacity

II. Answer the following questions in the space provided.

1. What are the two purposes of respiration?

2. Discuss seven factors that are necessary for proper oxygenation.

3. List four ways to maintain resistance to respiratory infection.

4. What are the three signs of a major pulmonary disorder?

5. What are three obstructive pulmonary disorders?

6. What breath sounds are heard when auscultating a patient with acute bronchitis?

7. Discuss the precautions when using a humidifier.

8. In what four states is tuberculosis most common?

9. List the guidelines for sputum specimen collection.

10. Discuss the etiology, signs and symptoms, and medical therapy for asthma.

III. Complete the following matching exercises.

A. Match the following medications with the desired effect.

a. Decrease secretions
b. Increase secretions
c. Depress cough reflex
d. Thin secretions

1. _____ Expectorants
2. _____ Anticholinergic agents
3. _____ Mucolytic agents
4. _____ Antitussives

B. Match the following lung volumes with the correct definition.

a. Maximal volume that can be inspired from the end of a normal inspiration
b. Total amount of air in lung after maximal inspiration (TV + IRV + ERV + RV)
c. Volume of gas inspired and expired with a normal breath
d. Maximal volume that can be exhaled by forced expiration after a normal expiration
e. Volume of gas left in lung after maximal expiration
f. Maximal amount of air that can be expired after a maximal inspiration (TV + IRV + ERV)
g. Maximal amount of air that can be expelled with a maximal effort after a maximal inspiration

1. _____ Tidal volume
2. _____ Inspiratory reserve volume
3. _____ Expiratory reseve volume
4. _____ Residual volume
5. _____ Vital capacity
6. _____ Total lung capacity

IV. Multiple choice

1. The process of respiration occurs only in:
a. Lungs **c.** Alveoli
b. Capillaries **d.** Bronchioles

2. Gas exchange within the pulmonary system from the blood occurs through:
a. Osmosis **c.** Active transport
b. Diffusion **d.** Oncotic pressure

3. What part of the brain can consciously control respiratory rate?
a. The pons **c.** Cerebral cortex
b. Medulla **d.** Chemoreceptors

4. The signs and symptoms of carbon monoxide poisoning are headache, lethargy, and tachycardia. These initial reactions to hypoxia are very similar to what a person experiences:
a. Under anesthesia **c.** With some drugs
b. At high altitudes **d.** Under stress

5. An example of a chronic obstructive lung disease is:
a. Tuberculosis **c.** Atelectasis
b. Pulmonary fibrosis **d.** Chronic bronchitis

6. The color of productive sputum is important in respiratory assessment. What is the color of sputum when a patient has staphylococcal pneumonia?
a. Greenish **c.** Yellowish
b. Creamy **d.** Rusty

7. The Mantoux test is performed to diagnose tuberculosis. It is important that the test be read:
a. Within 24 hours **c.** Within 48 to 72 hours
b. Within 48 hours **d.** Within 3 to 4 days

8. Which of the following interpretations of the Mantoux test is correct?
   a. 4 mm indicates probability of tuberculosis
   b. 0 mm indicates test did not take
   c. 5 mm is diagnostic for tuberculosis
   d. 10 mm is highly significant for infection
9. Which instructions would result in the best sputum specimen?
   a. "Take a deep breath and hold it. Cough. Now spit into this container."
   b. "Limit the amount of fluids you drink today. Tomorrow you will need to collect whatever you cough up in this container."
   c. "Spit whatever sputum you have in your mouth into this container."
   d. "Cough and deep breathe first thing tomorrow morning and collect whatever you cough up. Now practice coughing."
10. When the patient is on a ventilator, lungs are auscultated every hour to assess placement of the endotracheal tube. Why is this necessary?
    a. It can slip out of place when the patient turns
    b. When the patient coughs, it can pull back up
    c. It could slip into right mainstream bronchus
    d. It could become detached from balloon
11. Mrs. Miller is prepared for a diagnostic test. The nurse explains, "The test you'll be having in the morning allows the doctor to view your trachea and bronchi by inserting an instrument down your throat." The nurse has partially explained which diagnostic test?
    a. Bronchoscopy
    b. Bronchogram
    c. Computerized tomography
    d. Pulmonary angiography
12. The ability of the lungs to stretch to accommodate for increase in volume is called:
    a. Pressure
    b. Compliance
    c. Resistance
    d. Exchange
13. Which of the following lung surgeries does not require chest tubes?
    a. Lobectomy
    b. Pneumonectomy
    c. Segmental resection
    d. Wedge resection
14. A chest tube is necessary and is connected to water-sealed drainage. The purpose of this treatment is to restore what pressure in the pleural space?
    a. Atmospheric pressure
    b. Balanced pressure
    c. Negative pressure
    d. Positive pressure
15. What is the correct placement of the distal tip of the chest tube in the drainage bottle?
    a. Just below the bottle stopper
    b. 1 to 2 cm above the water level
    c. 1 to 2 cm below the water level
    d. 4 to 6 cm below the water level
16. Paradoxical respiratory movement, severe chest pain, and tachypnea with shallow respirations are signs of:
    a. Flail chest
    b. Hypercapnia
    c. Pneumothorax
    d. Heart attack
17. Which of the following is used as a measurement to determine adequate ventilation and the ability of the lungs to eliminate carbon dioxide?
    a. PaO_2
    b. $PaCO_2$
    c. Blood pH
    d. Ions
18. Hypoventilation results in which respiratory complication?
    a. Pneumonia
    b. Atelectasis
    c. Respiratory alkalosis
    d. Respiratory acidosis
19. A "barrel chest" is a sign of what disorder:
    a. Acute bronchitis
    b. Lung cancer
    c. Flail chest
    d. Emphysema

20. Which of the following assessment data is indicative of an abnormal finding upon inspection during a pulmonary examination?
    a. Inspiration/expiration ratio of 1:2
    b. Leans forward with hands on knees
    c. Skin translucent, mucous membranes moist
    d. Quiet respirations at rate of 20
21. What type of breathing is encouraged for the person with chronic obstructive pulmonary disease?
    a. Increase rate within comfortable limits
    b. Open mouth during inspiration
    c. Purse lips during expiration
    d. Increase time of inspiration
22. Asthma differs from bronchitis and emphysema because it:
    a. Is a restrictive lung disease
    b. Occurs only in children
    c. Has intermittent airway obstruction
    d. Has permanent airway blockage
23. The onset of an asthmatic attack is usually:
    a. Sudden with cough and hemoptysis
    b. Slow with gradual rise in temperature
    c. Slow with increasing dyspnea
    d. Sudden with coughing and wheezing
24. On auscultation the nurse hears a continuous, low-pitched sound. What abnormal sound has been identified?
    a. Crackles
    b. Rhonchi
    c. Wheeze
    d. Friction rub
25. The patient begins to cough during suctioning. What is the best nursing action?
    a. Auscultate lung sound
    b. Continue suctioning mucus
    c. Discontinue suctioning to allow for cough
    d. Position patient in the supine position
26. Which intervention before suctioning will decrease hypoxia during suctioning?
    a. Ambu breathe with 100% oxygen
    b. Lubricate suction catheter
    c. Suction for only 25 to 30 seconds
    d. Use a small catheter to suction
27. When suctioning the respiratory tract, the nurse should limit suctioning to periods of:
    a. 3 to 5 seconds
    b. 10 to 15 seconds
    c. 15 to 20 seconds
    d. 20 to 25 seconds
28. If suctioning must be repeated, it is recommended that the nurse wait at least 3 minutes. This is to allow time for:
    a. Overcoming fatigue
    b. Numbing of mucous membrane
    c. Replenishing of oxygen
    d. Subsiding of pain

V. Complete the following exercises.

1. Write the nursing interventions when caring for a patient with ARDS.
2. Write the nursing interventions for maintaining chest tubes and closed chest drainage.
3. Write a nursing care plan for a patient with COPD.
4. Write a nursing care plan for a patient on mechanical ventilation with PEEP.

SUGGESTED READINGS

Buckingham, AK: Arterial blood gases made simple, Nurs Life 5:48-51, Nov/Dec 1985.
An explanation of the components of ABGs, normal values, and how to interpret the report.

Carroll, PF: What you can learn from pulmonary function tests, RN 49:24-27, July 1986.
Identifies components of pulmonary function tests (PFTs), how to use the results to differentiate between restriction and obstructive lung disease, and how to coordinate medications and PFTs.

Coleman, DA: TB: the disease that's not dead yet, RN 47:48-57, Sept 1984.
The author dscribes how a person contracts TB, how it progresses, risk factors, diagnostic tests, drugs used in its treatment. Also provided is an in-depth description of skin tests. The author also tells when to isolate the TB patient, what to teach the patient, and how TB can be controlled.

Cross, M: Dissolving the threat of pulmonary embolism, RN 47:34-39, Aug 1984.
Through use of a case study, the author describes how PE begins, assessment findings, risk factors, and appropriate interventions.

D'Agostino, JS: Teaching tips for living with COPD, Nursing 14:57, Feb 1984.
The author describes things to do to minimize the spread of dust when house cleaning, such as dusting with a damp cloth, what to keep room temperature during the day and night, how to remove allergens and irritants from the house in the bedroom, bathroom, and kitchen.

Hahn, AB, and others: Chapters 26, 27, 28, 36 in Mosby's pharmacology in nursing, ed 17, St Louis, 1986, The CV Mosby Co.

Heggie, J and Chang M: What to do about flu, RN 46:60-63, Jan 1983.
The etiology, transmission, clinical manifestations, prevention, and nursing care for influenza is described. Information about vaccination, associated risks, and persons who should be vaccinated against the flu is provided.

Rifas, EM: Teaching patients to manage acute asthma: the future is now, Nursing 13:77-82, Apr 1983.
Through a case study the author describes the clinical manifestations, precipitating factors in an asthma attack, diagnostic tests, how to prevent an attack, and what patient assessments to make during an attack. Also described are the treatment and how to teach the patient to use the metered-dose inhalers.

Taylor, DL: Respiratory acidosis: physiology, signs, and symptoms, Nursing 14:44-45, Oct 1984.
A brief description of causes, clinical findings associated with underlying physiological changes in respiratory acidosis, and how the kidneys compensate.

Taylor, DL: Respiratory alkalosis: physiology, signs, and symptoms, Nursing 14:44-45, Nov 1984.
A brief description of causes, clinical findings associated with underlying physiological changes in respiratory alkalosis, and how the kidneys compensate.

Wimsatt, R: Unlocking the mysteries behind the chest wall, Nursing 15:58-63, Nov 1985.
A review of chest assessment using observation, palpation, percussion, and auscultation. Diagram showing anterior and posterior landmarks of the chest. Through use of short case studies of patients with COPD and heart disease, the authors describe how to peform a chest assessment.

Chapter 25

The Patient with Cardiovascular Problems

MARY S. NICHOLS

CHAPTER OBJECTIVES

On completion of this chapter, the student should be able to:

- Differentiate between data obtained from a 12-lead ECG and data obtained from a cardiac monitor.
- Explain the differences between arrhythmias that are a disturbance of impulse initiation and those of impulse conduction, and identify life-threatening arrhythmias.
- Describe treatment modalities for cardiac arrhythmias.
- Identify risk factors for CAD.
- Explain the pathophysiologic basis, therapeutic modalities, and nursing interventions for angina pectoris and myocardial infarction, and congestive heart failure.
- Identify teaching needs of patients with angina, myocardial infarction, and congestive heart failure, and patients undergoing cardiac surgery.
- Describe the pathophysiologic bases for pulmonary edema and cardiogenic shock; relate the therapeutic modalities for these conditions to those for congestive heart failure.
- Explain the pathophysiologic bases for disorders of the various layers of cardiac tissue (pericardium, myocardium, epicardium), the cardiac valves, and the aorta.
- Describe surgical intervention for repair of cardiac valves and aortic aneurysms and the pre/postoperative nursing care required.

PREREQUISITE READING

Long-Phipps, Chapter 25, p. 755-824.

SELF-ASSESSMENT ACTIVITIES

I. Define the following terms.

Alcoholic myopathy
Ambu bag
Aneurysms
Angina pectoris
Angiographic studies
Arrhythmia
Arteriosclerosis
Asystole
Atherosclerosis
Atrial fibrillation
Atrial flutter
Atrial 'kick'
AV block
AV node
Bacterial endocarditis
Carbohydrate intolerance
Cardiac output
Cardiogenic shock
Congestive heart failure
Coronary angioplasty
Coronary artery bypass surgery
Coronary artery disease
Counterpulsation
CVP
Dyspnea on exertion
Edema
Heparinization
Holter monitor
Hyperkinetic pulse
Hyperlipoproteinemia
Hypokinetic pulse
Inflammatory heart disease
Immunosuppression
MCL
Myocardial oxygen demand
Palpitations
Paroxysmal nocturnal dyspnea
PAT
Percutaneous transluminal coronary angioplasty
Pulsus alternans
Pulsus paradoxus dyspnea
PVB
SA node
Serum cholesterol
Serum enzymes

Continued

Sinus bradycardia	Stroke volume	Thrombocytopenia
Sinus tachycardia	Supraventricular tachycardia	Ventricular fibrillation
Stenotic heart disease	Telemetry	Ventricular tachycardia

II. Identification

1. Label the parts of the heart on the diagram below.
2. Draw arrows to show the flow of blood from the general circulation through the heart and then back to the general circulation.

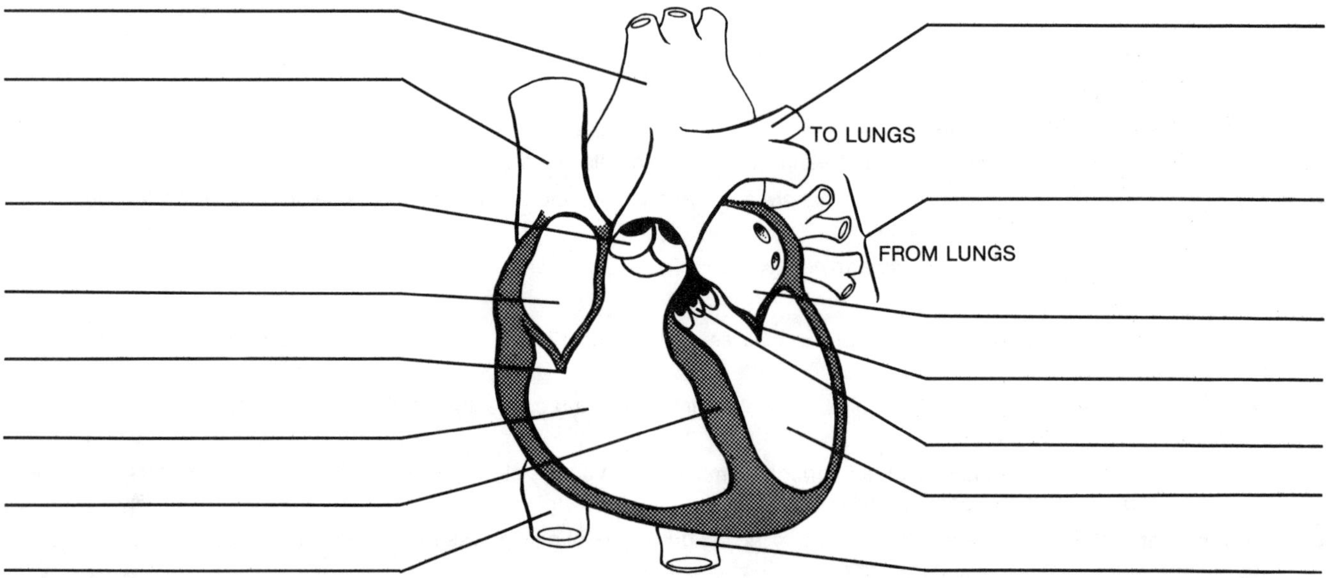

III. Answer the following questions in the space provided.

1. How much fluid is contained in the pericardial space? What is the primary function of this fluid?

2. What is the primary function of the coronary arteries?

3. What is the average cardiac output in the average adult?

4. What are the three factors that control stroke volume?

5. What is the major impedance against which the left ventricle must pump?

6. What is the primary determinant of preload?

IV. Multiple choice

1. During which phase of the cardiac cycle does coronary artery blood flow to the myocardium occur?
   - **a.** Diastole
   - **b.** Systole
2. During diastole:
   - **a.** The ventricles contract
   - **b.** The AV valves open
   - **c.** The aortic and pulmonic valves open
   - **d.** Systolic blood pressure is obtained
3. When hypertension occurs:
   - **a.** Afterload increases
   - **b.** Afterload decreases
   - **c.** Preload remains unchanged
   - **d.** Preload increases
4. Contractility of the heart muscle:
   - **a.** Is increased by sympathetic stimulation
   - **b.** Is decreased by calcium
   - **c.** Facilitates ventricular filling
   - **d.** Decreases stroke volume
5. Stimulation of baroreceptors in the carotid sinus or aortic arch:
   - **a.** Decreases blood pressure
   - **b.** Increases body temperature
   - **c.** Causes decreased heart rate
   - **d.** Causes increased heart rate
6. Which of the following factors reduces efficiency of the heart as a pump in aging persons?
   - **a.** Decreased amounts of connective tissue in heart muscle
   - **b.** Increased elasticity of aorta and major arteries
   - **c.** Endocardial sclerosis, thickening and fibrosis

V. Arrange the terms below to show the sequence of impulse transmission through the conduction system of the heart.

Bundle of His
AV node
Purkinje's fibers
SA node
right and left Bundle branches

VI. Compare central cyanosis with peripheral cyanosis.

	Central cyanosis	**Peripheral cyanosis**
Cause		
Manifestations		

VII. Label the components of the ECG wave on the diagram below using the symbols below.

T	S-T segment
P	QRS complex
Q	U wave
R	QT interval
S	

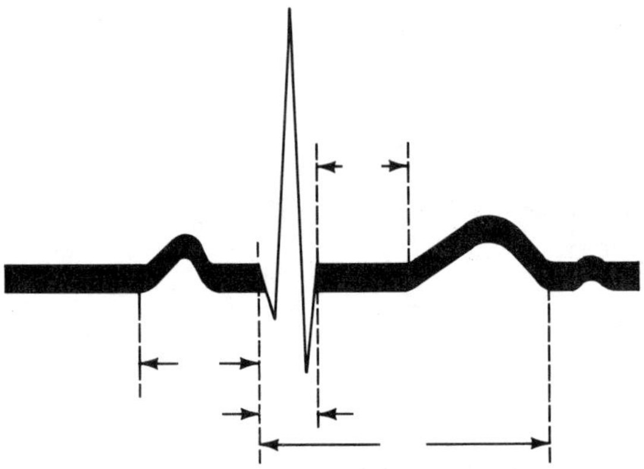

VIII. Complete the crossword puzzle on p. 149.

ACROSS

1. The difference between systolic and diastolic pressure
2. The middle layer of the heart
3. HR x SV equals
4. Outer layer of the heart
5. The ability of the heart to initiate impulses regularly and spontaneously
6. A type of murmur that occurs between S_2 and S_1
7. Dyspnea in the recumbent position
8. The ability of cardiac cells to respond to a stimulus by initiating a cardiac impulse

DOWN

1. CO x R equals
3. The ability of the heart to respond to an impulse by transmitting the impulse along cell membranes
9. Inner most layer of the heart
10. The volume of blood distending the ventricles at the end of diastole
11. Muscular wall which divides heart into two halves
12. Amount of tension the ventricles must develop in order to eject blood from the left ventricle into the aorta
13. A type of murmur that occurs between S_1 and S_2
14. Type of blood lipid that has the lowest athrogenic potential

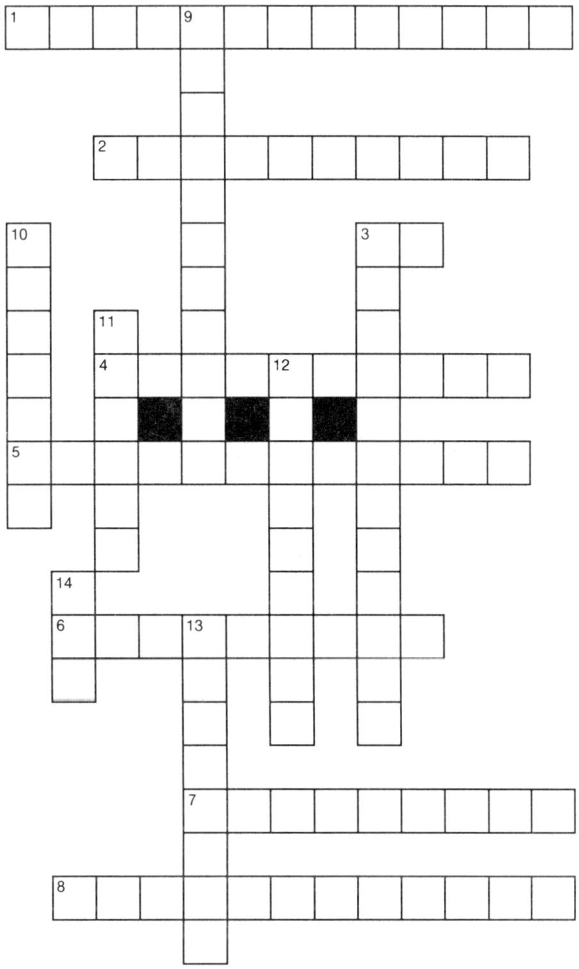

IX. Match the ECG configurations listed with the appropriate description below.

a. P wave
b. QRS complex
c. T wave
d. PR interval
e. S-T segment
f. QT interval

1. _____ Represents the entire duration of ventricular contraction
2. _____ Represents the final phase of ventricular repolarization
3. _____ Represents atria depolarization
4. _____ Represents the early phase of ventricular repolarization
5. _____ Represents the amount of time taken for the impulse to travel from the SA node to the ventricles
6. _____ Represents depolarization of the ventricles

X. The figure below shows a normal ECG configuration and normal values for ECG intervals. (PR interval 0.12 to 0.20 sec. QRS duration should not exceed 0.11 sec.) Using the ECG, identify the arrhythmia and answer the questions in the space provided.

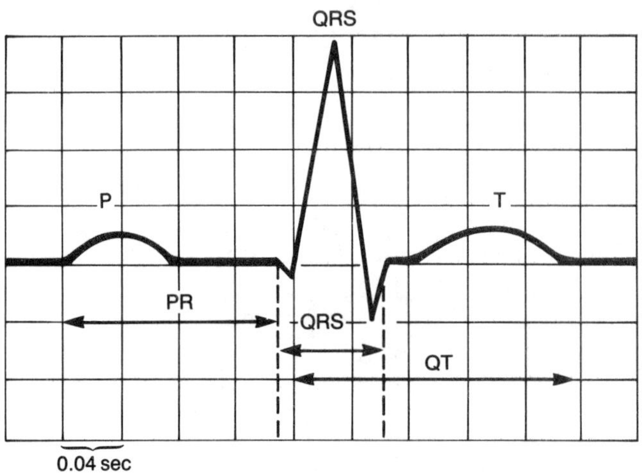

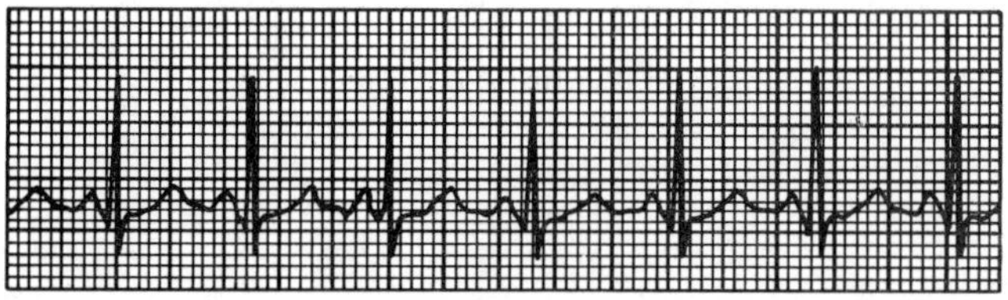

1. What is the heart rate? ______________ (Count the number of large blocks between an R-R interval. Then, divide the number of large blocks into 300.)

2. What is the PR interval?

3. What is the QRS interval?

4. Is the rhythm regular or irregular? (Measures the R-R intervals. If they are the same then the rhythm is regular.)

5. Are P waves present?

6. Is there a P wave for every QRS complex?

7. What is the arrhythmia?
   - **a.** Sinus arrhythmia
   - **b.** Sinus tachycardia
   - **c.** Sinus bradycardia
   - **d.** Sick sinus syndrome

XI. Multiple choice

1. Arrhythmias arise from disturbances in:
- **a.** Rate and rhythm
- **b.** Contractility and cardiac output
- **c.** Automaticity and conductivity
- **d.** Cardiac output and circulation

2. Sinus arrhythmia:
- **a.** Must be treated with a temporary pacemaker
- **b.** Generally requires defibrillation
- **c.** Generally requires cardioversion
- **d.** Is a benign arrhythmia that requires no treatment

3. Which of the following statements about sinus tachycardia is incorrect?
- **a.** The P waves are ventricular in origin.
- **b.** It is a benign rhythm.
- **c.** Patients may complain of palpitations.
- **d.** It is associated with ingestion of stimulants and exercise.

4. Sinus bradycardia:
- **a.** Can be caused by increased vagal stimulation
- **b.** Must be treated with cardioversion
- **c.** Is a life-threatening arrhythmia
- **d.** Is associated with excess use of caffeine or tobacco products

5. Which of the following drugs may be used to correct severe sinus bradycardia?
- **a.** Digoxin
- **b.** Levophed
- **c.** Atropine
- **d.** Aramine

6. When the term "sinus" is used in connection with an arrhythmia, it means that:
- **a.** The arrhythmia is caused by sinusitis
- **b.** The atria are contracting prematurely
- **c.** The impulse originated in the AV node
- **d.** The impulse originated in the SA node

7. Treatment for atrial fibrillation may include all *except:*
- **a.** Defibrillation
- **b.** Cardioversion
- **c.** Administration of digitalis
- **d.** Administration of propranolol

8. Which atrial arrhythmia is characterized by the presence of a sawtooth pattern of rapid atrial activity?
- **a.** Flutter
- **b.** Fibrillation
- **c.** Paroxysmal atrial tachycardia
- **d.** Premature atrial contraction

9. The major physiological alteration that causes symptoms in patients with persistent arrhythmias, regardless of the type, is:
- **a.** Hypercoagulability of the blood
- **b.** Decreased cardiac output
- **c.** Increased peripheral vascular resistance
- **d.** Cardiac standstill

10. On assessment of the patient with atrial fibrillation, the nurse would expect to find all *except:*
- **a.** Pulse deficit
- **b.** Irregular pulse
- **c.** Heart murmur
- **d.** No identifiable P waves on the ECG strip

11. A wide bizarre QRS complex is the most outstanding characteristic of which arrhythmia?
    a. Premature ventricular contractions
    b. Atrial flutter
    c. First degree heart block
    d. Paroxysmal atrial tachycardia
12. The severity of AV block is identified by:
    a. The extent of ventricular compensation
    b. Whether loss of consciousness occurs
    c. Whether hypotension occurs
    d. Degrees
13. The intensity of the electrical impulse delivered by the pulse generator of a cardiac pacemaker is:
    a. Measured in kilowatts
    b. Set at the lowest level that will produce depolarization
    c. Set at the highest level that will produce repolarization
    d. Determined by the patients level of activity

XII. Indicate which type of pacemaker can be used to stimulate the heart chambers below.

T = Temporary   P = Permanent

1. _____ Stimulation of ventricles only
2. _____ Stimulation of atria only
3. _____ Synchronous stimulation of both atria and ventricles

XIII. Write your answers in the space provided.

1. What is the greatest hazard associated with the use of asynchronous (fixed rate) pacing?

2. When is cardioversion indicated in the treatment of arrhythmias?

3. What is the primary difference between cardioversion and defibrillation?

4. What drug is used to treat arrhythmias that have been caused by digitalis toxicity?

5. What arrhythmia is treated by applying carotid sinus pressure or vagal stimulation?

6. What is the treatment for ventricular tachycardia? For ventricular fibrillation?

7. What is the most classic characteristic of:
   Right bundle branch block

   Left bundle branch block

XIV. Complete the chart below to compare the different atrioventricular blocks.

	First degree	Second degree		Third degree
		Mobitz I	Mobitz II	
Most outstanding ECG features				
Associated conditions				
Treatment				

XV. Complete the following chart for coronary artery disease.

Disease definition	CAHD	Angina pectoris	Myocardial infarction	Cardiogenic shock
Epidemiology				
Pathophysiology				
Modifiable risk factors				
Nonmodifiable risk factors				
Diagnoses				
Medical management				
Surgical management				
Patient teaching				

XVI. Complete the chart below on dynamic studies of the cardiovascular system.

	Holter monitor
Indications for use	
What to tell the patient	
Stress testing	
Definition	
Indications for use	
What test involves	
What is involved in patient preparation	
Manifestations of an abnormal stress test	

XVII. Complete the following chart.

Disease/etiology	**Pathophysiology**	**Clinical manifestation**	**Diagnostic tests**
Acute pericarditis			
Chronic pericarditis			
Myocarditis			
Alcoholic myopathy			

Continued

Disease/etiology	Pathophysiology	Clinical manifestation	Diagnostic tests
Infective endocarditis			
Rheumatic heart disease			
Syphilitic heart disease			

XVIII. Completion

A. Complete the following chart on valvular heart disease (review text).

Type of valvular disease	Pathophysiology	Clinical manifestations	Interventions
Mitral valvular disease			
Mitral regurgitation			
Aortic valvular disease			
Tricuspid valvular disease			
Pulmonic valvular disease			

B. List the nursing interventions related to each valvular disease.

Mitral valvular disease

Mitral regurgitation

Aortic valvular disease

Tricuspid valvular disease

Pulmonic valvular disease

XIX. Multiple choice

1. Modifiable rise factors for coronary atherosclerotic heart disease include all but one of the following:
   - **a.** Psychologic stress
   - **b.** Race, age, sex
   - **c.** Hypertension and smoking
   - **d.** Obesity
2. Which statement is true about coronary atherosclerosis?
   - **a.** It is caused by stiffening of arteries.
   - **b.** Its cause is unknown.
   - **c.** Its presence is immediately detectable.
   - **d.** Young adults do not have this pathologic condition.
3. Angina pectoris is relieved by:
   - **a.** Rest
   - **b.** Vasoconstriction
   - **c.** Vasodilation
   - **d.** Analgesics
4. The nurse who is discharging a patient should give instructions regarding nitroglycerin administration for pain. Which is the most appropriate statement?
   - **a.** If the pain is not relieved after three doses of nitroglycerin, have your spouse call the ambulance. Pain may be caused by a heart attack.
   - **b.** Keep a supply of oxygen at home to administer if pain is not relieved.
   - **c.** Call your physician if pain is not relieved after three doses.
   - **d.** Take another dose of nitroglycerin if pain is not relieved after three doses.
5. The purpose of coronary artery bypass is to:
   - **a.** Lengthen life
   - **b.** Lessen the possibility of myocardial infarction
   - **c.** Modify atherosclerosis
   - **d.** Increase myocardial supply of oxygen
6. Percutaneous transluminal coronary angioplasty:
   - **a.** Is a mechanical dilation of a coronary vessel wall
   - **b.** Is a procedure that usually precedes coronary bypass surgery
   - **c.** Is done to remove atheromatous plaques
   - **d.** Usually requires only 1 day of hospitalization
7. Which of the following decreases myocardial oxygen demand?
   - **a.** Bed rest
   - **b.** O_2 by nasal cannula
   - **c.** Morphine sulfate IV
   - **d.** Lidocaine IV
8. In mild cardiac failure, the most effective method of assisting a patient to reduce fluid retention is to:
   - **a.** Reduce fluid intake
   - **b.** Add herbs and garlic
   - **c.** Follow diet prescription for salt
   - **d.** Increase cardiac output
9. If rotating tourniquets are prescribed to reduce cardiac overload, they should be placed on three limbs and:
   - **a.** Should be rotated every 15 minutes
   - **b.** Each extremity is occluded for 30 minutes
   - **c.** Should obliterate femoral arteries
   - **d.** Should be removed from arms first
10. For a patient who has alcoholic myopathy, a nurse should suggest:
    - **a.** That the patient should limit alcohol intake
    - **b.** Alcoholics Anonymous can help the patient abstain for life
    - **c.** That the enlargement of the patient's heart can be reversed by moderation
    - **d.** That the patient modify his or her diet

11. Cardiac pain caused by congestive heart failure is usually a result of:
    a. Dyspnea
    b. Anxiety
    c. Cough
    d. Angina pectoris
12. The positive inotropic action of digitalis enhances the mechanical function of the heart. Which other property affects the heart rate?
    a. Conductivity
    b. Automaticity
    c. Contractility
    d. Tonicity
13. Which of the following are *not* indicators of digitalis toxicity?
    a. Double vision, confusion, and drowsiness
    b. Nausea, vomiting, diarrhea
    c. Increased urinary output and adequate potassium
    d. Cardiac arrhythmias
14. What is the acceptable time period for apical pulse measurement before administration of digoxin?
    a. 30 seconds
    b. 60 seconds
    c. 15 seconds
    d. 10 seconds
15. What should be done by the nurse if the pulse rate is 52 before administering digoxin?
    a. Administer the drug and notify the physician
    b. Notify physician
    c. Withhold the drug, notify physician
16. The key to reassessing administration of diuretics is:
    a. Hypotension
    b. Reduced urinary output
    c. Increased urinary output
    d. Hypertension
17. Another group of drugs used to treat acute congestive heart failure is the:
    a. Antilipidemics
    b. Anticoagulants
    c. Vasodilators
    d. Vasoconstrictors
18. Before administration of diuretics, which of the following should be done daily?
    a. Weight noted
    b. Vital signs taken
    c. Peripheral pulse assessment
    d. Assessment for edema
19. Which of the following is a desired outcome for a person with congestive heart failure include?
    a. The person can plan his or her own diet.
    b. The person can return to work.
    c. The person's breathing is easier.
    d. The person states he will visit his physician after discharge.

XX. Complete the list below and on p. 158 for abdominal aortic aneurysms. List the following major points of content in reference to aneurysms.

Etiology

Pathophysiology

Diagnostic tests

Nursing assessment

Postoperative care

Discharge instructions

XXI. Complete the list below for open heart surgery.

Preoperative care

Procedure

Intraortic balloon counterpulsation (IABP)

Postoperative assessment of major systems

Support of fluid and electrolyte balance

Comfort, rest and sleep

Psychologic response

Activity

Patient teaching

SUGGESTED READINGS

Boyd MD, and Citro KM: "Is your MI patient too scared to recover? RN 51:50-54, May 1988.
The rehabilitation of the MI patient begins in the ED, teaching patients how to relax and helping the patient cope with preparation for discharge. An insert describes an exercise regimen.

Klein, D: Angina—pathophysiology and resulting signs and symptoms, Nurs 88 18(7):28-31, 1988.
Graphic colored drawings illustrate angina syndrome, pathophysiology, and assessments and intervention.

Morris, LL: Critical care's most versatile tool . . . a multilumen central venous catheter (pictorial), RN 51(5):42-46, 1988.
The advantages of using triple-lumen IV catheter for continuous and intermittent use. Describes use of each lumen, equipment needed for insertion, and provides photo guide for administration of medications. Sterile site care to prevent infection is explained.

O'Malley, P: Relationship of hope and stress after myocardial infarction,

Smith, CE: Assessing chest pain quickly and accurately, Nurs 88 18(5):52-60, 1988.
CEU-approved article cites characteristics for analyzing symptoms, gathering of subjective and objective data, and provides an insert on minimizing the patient's anxiety; there is a flow diagram, care presentation, and a 23-item quiz.

Chapter 26

The Patient with Peripheral Vascular Problems

BRENDA GOODNER

CHAPTER OBJECTIVES

On completion of this chapter, the student should be able to:

- Identify risk factors associated with the development of peripheral vascular disorders.
- Describe pathophysiology, nursing diagnoses, expected outcomes, and interventions for patients with arterial and venous disorders.
- Describe nursing interventions for patients having surgery for arterial and venous disorders.
- Describe the pathophysiology and nursing interventions for patients with leg ulcers and lymph disorders.
- Describe the pathophysiology and nursing interventions for persons with hypertension.

PREREQUISITE READING

Long-Phipps, Chapter 26, pp. 825-861.

SELF-ASSESSMENT ACTIVITIES

I. Define the following terms.

Aneurysm
Arteriosclerosis obliterans
Atherosclerosis
Beta blockers
Diuretics
Endarterectomy
Hyperlipidemia
Hypertension
Intermittent claudication
Lymph nodes
Lymphedema
Malignant hypertension
Phantom limb pain
Primary prevention
Prosthesis
Renin-angiotensin system
Secondary prevention
Thrombophlebitis
Varicose veins
Vasodilators

II. Answer the following questions.

1. List seven risks factors associated with peripheral vascular disease.

2. The two most commonly prescribed anticoagulants are:

3. Explain the five steps in the use of elastic stockings.

4. List ten measures that can be taken to decrease lymphedema.

5. List ten nursing interventions when administering heparin.

6. What medication counteracts the anticoagulant effects of coumadin?

III. Match the diagnostic test to the appropriate explanation.

a. Arteriography (angiography)
b. Exercise testing
c. Doppler test
d. Digital subtraction angiography
e. Cold stimulation test

1. ______ Determines exercise that precipitates claudication
2. ______ Assessment of arterial blood flow
3. ______ Detection of deep-vein thrombophlebitis
4. ______ Used to diagnose Reynaud's phenomenon
5. ______ Visualization of vascular system to determine occlusion

IV. Complete the following chart on hypertension.

Type of hypertension	Risk factors or causes	Pathophysiology	Signs and symptoms
Essential (primary)			
Secondary			
Malignant hypertension			

V. Multiple choice

1. Venous thrombi tend to form in which of these locations:
   a. Bifurcations of superficial veins
   b. Valves
   c. Bifurcations of deep veins
   d. In the lung
2. Which intervention is recommended to promote tissue perfusion and comfort?
   a. Apply warm moist heat to affected extremity
   b. Perform range of motion to affected extremity
   c. Allow person's affected leg to dangle
   d. Discourage complete bed rest

3. Anticoagulants such as heparin or coumadin are often administered to a patient with peripheral vascular disease. The purpose of anticoagulants is:
   a. To thin blood so clots can flow easily
   b. To inhibit further clot formation
   c. To prevent buildup of RBCs in blood
   d. To prevent thrombus from breaking loose
4. The correct position for the patient with a below-the-knee amputation is:
   a. Low Fowler's with no flexion of hip or knee
   b. Flat with affected extremity elevated
   c. High Fowler's with extremity flat
   d. Semi-Fowler's with knee flexed with pillow
5. Mrs. Willis, 52, is a postsurgical patient complaining of pain in the calf of her leg. The nurse assesses warmth and redness in the area. Homan's sign is positive. This assessment is indicative of:
   a. Varicose veins
   b. Venous insufficiency
   c. Arterial occlusion
   d. Thrombophlebitis
6. Which of the following is an early symptom of early arteriosclerosis obliterans?
   a. Gnawing or burning pain at rest
   b. Intermittent claudication
   c. Chronically cold hands and feet
   d. Diminished or absent pulses proximal to observation
7. Which of the following arterial disorders does not respond to surgical sympathectomy?
   a. Thromboangiitis obliterans
   b. Arteriosclerosis obliterans
   c. Reynaud's phenomenon and disease
   d. Arteriovenous fistula
8. Intermittent claudication is defined as:
   a. A cramp in the calf that lasts 1 to 2 minutes after cessation of the exercise
   b. A brief, knife-like pain in the distal extremities
   c. A burning sensation in the finger tips when exposed to cold
   d. Continuous bilateral pains in the feet lasting 10 minutes
9. There is a strong relationship between Buerger's disease and
   a. Exposure to cold
   b. Cigarette smoking
   c. Genetic predisposition
   d. Intimal injury
10. Peripheral pulses are which of the following?
    a. Carotid, temporal, femoral, radial, popliteal
    b. Radial, carotid, popliteal, dorsalis pedis
    c. Dorsalis pedis, popliteal, radial, ulnar, posterior tibialis, femoral
    d. Popliteal, ulnar, temporal, carotid, radial
11. The appropriate nursing action when Homan's sign is present is:
    a. Elevate the leg and apply cold pack
    b. Elevate the leg and apply heating pad
    c. Apply TED hose to leg immediately
    d. Massage leg with soft, upward strokes
12. The largest single cause of peripheral vascular disease is:
    a. Diabetes
    b. Varicose veins
    c. Hypertension
    d. Renal disease
13. Initially, moderate hypertension is treated with:
    a. Medications and exercise
    b. Low-salt diet and weight loss
    c. Diuretics and potassium
    d. Loading dose of digitalis

14. The activation of the renin-angiotensin system contributes to hypertension to some extent. Basically, it causes:
    a. Vasoconstriction and increased intravascular volume
    b. Vasoconstriction and decreased intravascular volume
    c. Vasodilation and increased intravascular volume
    d. Vasodilation and decreased intravascular volume
15. Preventive measures for peripheral vascular disorders include:
    a. Avoid smoking
    b. Avoid hot weather
    c. Use a comfortable soft mattress
    d. Wear belts rather than suspenders
16. What is the major complication of thrombophlebitis?
    a. Hemorrhage
    b. Infection
    c. Ulceration
    d. Embolism
17. Vascular changes occurring with hypertension can be directly observed in what part of the body?
    a. Fingernails
    b. Retina
    c. Neck
    d. Legs

VI. Complete the teaching plan for a patient diagnosed as having essential hypertension.

Content	Patient teaching
Pathology of hypertension	
Medications	
Nutrition counseling	
Smoking cessation	
Exercise program	
Stress management	
General health maintenance	

SUGGESTED READINGS

Bourne, BA, and Kutcher, JL: Amputation—helping a patient face loss of a limb, RN 85:39-45, Feb 1985.
Case study of diabetic, middle-aged diabetic man; comprehensive preoperative instructions and exercise; diagrams of stump bandaging; coping with postoperative problems, rehabilitation, prostheses, and changed life-style.

Doyle, JE: Treatment modalities in peripheral vascular disease, NCNA 21:241-253, June 1986.
Discussion of medical management, risk factor modification, prophylasic, pharmacotherapy, surgery of peripherovascular system.

Herman, JA: Nursing assessment and diagnosis in patients with peripheral vascular disease, NCNA, 21:219-231, June 1986.

Lasoff, EM: When a teenager faces amputation, RN 48(2):44-45, 1985.
Help for you to assist teenager who faces amputation, acceptance of friends, threat to independence, lack of privacy in hospital.

Turner, JA: Nursing intervention in patient with peripheral vascular disease. NCNA 21:233-239, June 1986.
Further in-depth discussion of modification of risk factors, pain relief, and hypercholesterolemia.

Chapter 27

The Patient with Hematologic Problems

BRENDA GOODNER

CHAPTER OBJECTIVES

On completion of this chapter, the student should be able to:

- Differentiate among the functions of red blood cells, white blood cells, platelets, and the lymph system.
- Compare and contrast different types of anemia in terms of pathophysiology, assessment, and interventions.
- Contrast bone marrow aspiration and biopsy, and describe the related care.
- Explain the genetic factors of sickle cell disease and describe sickle cell crisis.
- Compare and contrast disorders of coagulation (thrombocytopenia, hemophilia, DIC).
- Differentiate among the four types of leukemia and describe therapeutic modalities and nursing interventions.
- Differentiate between Hodgkin's disease and non-Hodgkin's lymphomas and describe treatment modalities and nursing interventions.

PREREQUISITE READING

Long-Phipps, Chapter 27, pp. 863-899.

SELF-ASSESSMENT ACTIVITES

I. Define the following terms.

Anemia
Bone marrow biopsy
Chemotheraphy
Coagulation factors
Disseminated intravascular coagulation
Eosinophils
Erythrocytes
Erythropoiesis
Hematopoiesis
Hemophilia
Hodgkin's disease
Idiopathic thrombocytopenia purpura
Leukemia
Leukocytes
Lymphadenopathy
Lymphocytes
Monocytes
Multiple myeloma
Neutrophils
Platelets
Reticuloendothelial system

II. Answer the following questions.

1. What are the two components of the hematopoietic system?

2. What are the three major cell components of the blood?

3. What is the important function of the reticuloendothelial system?

4. List four causes of anemia.

5. List six food sources of iron.

III. Match the following common coagulation tests with the appropriate description.

a. Time required for solid clot to form (less sensitive test than PTT) 5 to 10 minutes
b. Evaluation of vascular and platelets factors—the time it takes for a small stab wound to stop bleeding—2 to 9 minutes
c. More sensitive test than PT to evaluate adequacy of intrinsic coagulation pathway (fibrin clot formation) 60 to 90 seconds
d. Indicates rapidity of blood clotting (indicative of adequacy of extrinsic coagulation pathway; factors I, II, V, VII, X) 10% as compared to control levels

1. _____ Bleeding time
2. _____ Clotting time
3. _____ Prothrombin time (PT)
4. _____ Partial thromboplastin time (PTT)

IV. Complete the following chart on the primary anemias.

Type of anemia	Etiology	Pathophysiology	Clinical manifestations	Management
Aplastic				
Hemolytic				
Thalassemia				
Sickle cell				
Hemolytic				
Iron-deficiency				
Megaloblastic				

V. Multiple choice

1. The white blood cells that serve as the primary defense against infection are:
a. Lymphocytes
b. Eosinophils
c. Neutrophils
d. Basophils

2. The sequence of basic steps in the coagulation process is:
a. Thrombin, prothrombin, fibrinogen, fibrin
b. Prothrombin, thrombin, fibrin, fibrinogen
c. Thrombin, prothrombin, fibrinogen, fibrin
d. Prothrombin, thrombin, fibrinogen, fibrin

3. Granulocytes, lymphocytes, and monocytes are all examples of:
a. Leukocytes
b. Erythrocytes
c. Platelets
d. Immunoglobulins

4. Persons with disorders of the white blood cells need to be especially protected from:
a. Fever
b. Infection
c. Bleeding
d. Stress

5. Acute blood loss can have several serious effects on the body. Serious consequences result when the loss is:
a. 100 ml
b. 300 ml
c. 500 ml
d. 1000 ml

6. In acute blood loss transfusion the therapy usually indicated is:
a. Packed red cells
b. Whole blood
c. Fresh plasma
d. Frozen plasma

7. Pernicious anemia results from the genetic lack of an intrinsic factor that interferes with absorption of what substance?
a. Folic acid
b. Iron
c. Vitamin B_{12}
d. Vitamin K

8. Hematologic diseases are often associated with skin problems. Petechiae and ecchymoses are seen in:
a. Iron-deficiency anemia
b. Pernicious anemia
c. Thrombocytopenia
d. Vitamin K deficiency

9. The most important nursing intervention to prevent hemorrhage in a person with thrombocytopenia is:
a. Prevent trauma and falling
b. Avoid catheterization
c. Test urine with Hemastix for blood
d. Maintain a clean environment

10. Hemophilia is a sex-linked, recessive mendelian trait transmitted by the female and affecting only males. In families having the hemophiliac trait, who can reproduce with any assurance that the disease will not be transmitted?
a. Males only
b. Females only
c. Unaffected males
d. Unaffected females

11. The patient with DIC is extremely ill. An important function of the nurse is to observe the patient for:
a. Fluid overload
b. Increase or decrease in bleeding
c. New bleeding episodes
d. Hemorrhage

12. Stewart is a pale, thin, acutely ill child of 6 years who is admitted to the hospital. The physician made a tentative diagnosis of acute leukemia, and ordered: CBC and urinalysis, bone marrow biopsy, mouth care, and high-protein diet. Which of the following symptoms would be most characteristic of acute leukemia?
a. Nervousness and irritability
b. Tendency to bruise easily
c. Absence of sweating and coarse dry skin
d. Urine of low specific gravity

13. The physician reports that the biopsy establishes the diagnosis of leukemia. What would the laboratory report indicate?
    a. Large numbers of immature white blood cells
    b. Large numbers of RBCs and platelets
    c. Large numbers of mature white blood cells
    a. A radical change in plasma neutrophils
14. What type of leukemia seen in adults is characterized by immature white blood cells and by normal or decreased WBC serum levels?
    a. Acute lymphocytic
    b. Acute myelogenous
    c. Chronic lymphocytic
    d. Chronic myelogenous
15. The factor that is basic to nursing the patient with leukemia is:
    a. Remissions of the disease happen in 50% of persons with leukemia
    b. An honest nurse-patient relationship must be established and maintained
    c. The patient should have knowledge of his drug regimen
    d. Prevention of infection
16. The most important prognostic indicator of Hodgkin's disease is:
    a. The age and sex of the person who has the disease
    b. The general health of the patient
    c. The stage of the disease at the time of diagnosis
    d. Which of the several kinds of the disease it is
17. Hodgkin's disease is a malignant disorder of:
    a. Lymph nodes
    b. Muscle tissue
    c. Nervous system
    d. Blood system

Choose the most appropriate statement to complete each item.

18. Persons having a bone marrow aspiration should be cautioned by the nurse to:
    a. Lie still, especially when they feel a burning sensation
    b. Take deep breaths and cough
    c. Raise their shoulders and heads
    d. Watch for bleeding at the site
19. The population most at risk for sickle cell anemia is:
    a. India
    b. Mediterranean
    c. Black American
    d. Caribbean
20. Family planning is an important part of patient teaching in sickle cell anemia. This is because the disease is:
    a. Communicable
    b. Genetic
    c. Contagious
    d. Infectious
21. The most common event in sickle cell disease is:
    a. Renal problems from infarction
    b. Ocular problems
    c. Vasoocclusive crises
    d. Pain in back and chest
22. Sickling of red blood cells is caused by:
    a. Abnormality of the protien fraction of Hb
    b. Fragile cell membranes
    c. Hypochromic red cells
    d. Deviation in the normal number or sequence of amino acids
23. The nurse teaching a patient who is receiving oral iron supplement should tell the patient:
    a. Take medication after meals
    b. Take medication with meals
    c. Take medication before meals
    d. That his stools will be green
24. The most common cause of functional platelet abnormalities is:
    a. Aspirin
    b. Corticosteroids
    c. Injury
    d. Overhydration

VI. Write a nursing care plan for the patient suffering a sickle cell crisis.

SUGGESTED READINGS

Griffin, J: Be prepared for the bleeding patient, Nurs 86 16:34-42, June 1986.

Thorough discussion of DIC, secondary to septicemia, signs and symptoms, laboratory diagnosis, high risk bleeding precautions, assessing for thrombi and hemorrhages, estimating blood counts. Thirty-item quiz and check your answers with the text.

King, NH: Controlling bleeding when the platelet count drops, RN 47:25-27, August 1984.

Lists drugs that can cause thrombocytopenia, factors that destroy, dilute, or decrease platelet production, assessment, steps to prevent bleeding, and control of bleeding.

The latest protocols for blood transfusions—Committee on Transfusion Practices—American Association of Blood Banks, Nurs 86 16:34-41, October 1986.

Most recent protocols for blood transfusions covering each step in transfusion, compatibility, special equipment, pretransfusion testing. Illustrated pathophysiology of hemolytic reaction, complications and details you need to know about other blood components transfusion. Twenty-item quiz; check your answers in text of the article. Well-illustrated article.

UNIT VII **Metabolic and Endocrine Problems**

Chapter 28

The Patient with Diabetes Mellitus

BRENDA GOODNER

CHAPTER OBJECTIVES

On completion of this chapter, the student should be able to:

- Differentiate between the two major types of diabetes mellitus (DM).
- Describe prevention and health education for DM.
- Explain the pathophysiologic bases for hyperglycemia, nonketotic coma, diabetic ketoacidosis, macrovascular and microvascular changes, neuropathy, and lower extremity changes.
- Identify assessment parameters of DM.
- Describe the dietary recommendations and systems for learning dietary requirements.
- Explain the role of exercise in DM.
- Describe medication regimens for DM.
- Describe therapy for correcting acute metabolic crisis.
- Explain the effect of surgery on the person with DM.
- Identify and describe the ten commandments of importance in teaching the patient with DM.

PREREQUISITE READING

Long-Phipps, Chapter 28, pp. 903-940.

SELF-ASSESSMENT ACTIVITIES

I. Define the following terms.

Diabetes mellitus (DM)
Diabetic ketoacidosis
Diabetic retinopathy
Fasting blood sugar
Food exchange
Gestational diabetes mellitus (GDM)
Glucagon
Gluconeogenesis
Glycogenolysis
Glycosuria
Hyperglycemia
Hyperosmolality
Hypoglycemia
Hypoglycemic agents
Insulin
Ketogenesis
Lipodystrophy
Lipolysis
Nephropathy
Neuropathy
Postprandial
Somogyi phenomenon

II. Answer the following questions.

1. What affect does insulin have on blood glucose levels?

2. List the five classifications and a brief description of diabetes mellitus.

3. Compare insulin dependent and non-insulin dependent diabetes mellitus.

4. Discuss the primary and secondary prevention of DM.

5. List the blood tests, procedures, and interpretations related to DM.

6. Name the four most common signs and symptoms of hypoglycemia.

7. List the five classic signs of hyperglycemia.

8. Name the two major crises of diabetes mellitus and the signs and symptoms of each.

9. What percentage of each of the following is recommended daily for the diabetic patient?

   Protein ______%
   Carbohydrates ______%
   Fats ______%

10. List four examples of water-soluble fiber.

11. List the six food groups in the food exchange system.

III. Match the type of insulin with peak of action.

a. 2-4 hours
b. 8-12 hours
c. 4-7 hours
d. 16-18 hours

1. ______ Regular
2. ______ Semilente
3. ______ NPH
4. ______ Ultralente

IV. Multiple choice

1. The nurse assumes an important role in the care of the patient with diabetes mellitus. Much of the patient teaching concerning diet, exercise, and medication is nursing responsibility. This is especially important because the outcome of the disease process for each individual depends on:
   a. Self-medication
   b. Self-management
   c. Diet and exercise
   d. Diet and medication
2. Who is at highest risk for type 2 diabetes mellitus?
   a. The 9-year-old boy whose father has type 2
   b. The 20-year-old man whose mother has type 2
   c. The 40-year-old woman who is 30 pounds overweight
   d. The 60-year-old man who is 30 pounds overweight
3. The most common classification of diabetes mellitus is:
   a. IGT
   b. GDM
   c. IDDM, type 1
   d. NIDDM, type 2
4. Patients with Type II diabetes mellitus tend to be resistant to ketoacidosis. However, they are most vulnerable during:
   a. The menstrual cycle
   b. Carbohydrate bingeing
   c. Periods of fasting
   d. Periods of excessive stress
5. The condition that results from a lack or deficiency of insulin is called:
   a. Hyperglycemia
   b. Hypoglycemia
   c. Ketoacidosis
   d. Insipidus
6. Diabetic ketoacidosis occurs when:
   a. There is a severe insulin deficiency
   b. There is partial renal shutdown
   c. There is a blood glucose over 200
   d. There is severe dehydration

Mr. Morgan, 68, is hospitalized with hyperglycemia, hyperosmolar, nonketotic coma.

7. The complication to monitor in Mr. Morgan's condition is:
   a. Hemorrhage
   b. Infection
   c. Pancreatitis
   d. Dehydration
8. Mr. Morgan may experience CNS dysfunction as a result of his condition. The nurse knows this is related to:
   a. Severe hypoxia
   b. Cellular dysfunction
   c. Intracellular fluid loss
   d. Extracellular fluid loss
9. Dietary recommendations for diabetics are established by:
   a. American Dietetics Association (ADA)
   b. American Diabetes Association (ADA)
   c. American Medical Association (AMA)
   d. American Heart Association (AHA)
10. Long-term therapy in diabetes focuses on:
    a. Cure
    b. Weight loss
    c. Prevention
    d. Diet control
11. Diabetes is the leading cause of blindness in this country. This condition is called:
    a. Diabetic nephropathy
    b. Diabetic retinopathy
    c. Diabetic neuropathy
    d. Retina detachment
12. The blindness is caused by:
    a. Hemorrhage
    b. Tiny lesions
    c. Scar tissue
    d. Retina detachment
13. A complication that is closely related to diabetic retinopathy and should be carefully monitored is:
    a. Neuropathy
    b. Nephropathy
    c. Hypertension
    d. Hypotension

14. Neuropathy is a common disorder in diabetes. The most common neuropathy is symmetrical peripheral polyneuropathy. The early symptom of this complication is:
    - a. Difficulty with vision
    - b. Loss of multiple sensory functions
    - c. Numbness, tingling in extremities
    - d. Sensory loss in lower extremities
15. When ketone bodies are present in the blood and in the urine, it indicates faulty metabolism of:
    - a. Glucose
    - b. Amino acids
    - c. Fatty acids
    - d. Glycogen
16. Teaching a diabetic patient about foot care, should include instruction to:
    - a. Apply alcohol after cleansing feet
    - b. Check feet weekly
    - c. Wear socks with shoes at all times
    - d. Cut toenails close to the skin
17. In doing community health care, the best intervention to plan to decrease the incidence of diabetes would be:
    - a. Development of preventive health classes designed to decrease the incidence of obesity
    - b. Promotion of tissue typing to identify persons with histocompatibility complexes associated with diabetes
    - c. Development of genetic counseling clinics for use with couples anticipating starting a family
    - d. Development of screening clinics for screening for autoimmune disease
18. A serious complication of sensory neuropathy is:
    - a. Numbness, tingling
    - b. Diabetic foot
    - c. Loss of smell
    - d. Hearing impairment
19. The key to care of the diabetic foot is:
    - a. Medication
    - b. Self-care
    - c. Warm soaks
    - d. Do not trim nails
20. The action of all insulins is:
    - a. Hyperglycemic
    - b. Hypoglycemic
    - c. Hypertensive
    - d. Antagonistic
21. A bottle of insulin is labeled U-100. This means there are:
    - a. 100 units per dose
    - b. 100 units in the bottle
    - c. 100 mg per unit
    - d. 100 units per milliliter
22. In administering insulin it is essential that the insulin concentrations on the bottle match:
    - a. The insulin syringe calibration
    - b. A 3 ml (cc) syringe calibration
    - c. A syringe with 1 ml (cc)
    - d. The standard syringe calibration
23. After insulin is injected, it takes some time for it to take effect. The period of time at which it has the strongest effect is the:
    - a. Onset
    - b. Peak
    - c. Duration
    - d. Limit
24. A diabetic patient must carefully plan exercise around diet and medication. The patient must be constantly aware that exercise has:
    - a. A hyperglycemic effect
    - b. A cardiorespiratory effect
    - c. A hypoglycemic effect
    - d. A hypertensive effect
25. The complications of diabetes mellitus, diabetic ketoacidosis, and hyperglycemia, hyperosmolar, nonketoic coma can lead to shock, coma, and death. The major difference between DKA and HHNC is:
    - a. Death is much faster in DKA
    - b. Ketosis and acidosis is not seen in HHNC
    - c. DKA is seen in the elderly and HHNC in the young
    - d. HHNC is intracellular and DKA is extracellular
26. A common vascular complication of diabetes mellitus is:
    - a. Atherosclerosis
    - b. Phlebitis
    - c. Hypotension
    - d. Lactic acidosis

27. The term diabetic nephropathy refers to:
    - **a.** CNS functioning
    - **b.** Renal functioning
    - **c.** Liver functioning
    - **d.** Pancreatic functioning
28. At the onset clinical signs and symptoms of diabetic nephropathy are usually not seen. This abnormality is identified by:
    - **a.** Biopsy
    - **b.** Bone scan
    - **c.** X-ray
    - **d.** Blood test
29. Exercise for the diabetic is recommended when blood sugar is highest. This is:
    - **a.** 30 minutes after a meal
    - **b.** One hour after a meal
    - **c.** One to three hours after a meal
    - **d.** One hour before the next meal
30. The first-line treatment for hypoglycemia is:
    - **a.** Insulin injection
    - **b.** Simple carbohydrates
    - **c.** Glucagon injection
    - **d.** Complex carbohydrates
31. Hypoglycemia is caused by:
    - **a.** Excess sugar intake
    - **b.** Lack of exercise
    - **c.** Insulin excess
    - **d.** Too much exercise

V.

1. Write a teaching plan for an exercise program for a diabetic patient.

2. Discuss the major guidelines for administering insulin.

3. Discuss the Somogyi phenomenon.

SUGGESTED READINGS

McFadden, H: The ups and downs of diabetes, Am J Nurs 85:881-883, Aug 1985.
Graphic chart with symptoms of hypoglycemia and hyperglycemia.

McCarthy, JA: The continuation of diabetic coma, Am J Nurs 85:879-881, Aug 1985.
Case studies with discussion of persons with hypoglycemic coma, diabetic ketoacidosis and HHNK coma.

Teaching your patient about blood glucose testing, Nursing Life 5:41 Nov/Dec 1985.
Excellent summary for advantages of blood glucose testing over urine testing, gives examples when glucose testing is not required. Describes equipment needed. Line drawing of step-by-step self-testing.

Chapter 29

The Patient with Endocrine Problems

BRENDA GOODNER

CHAPTER OBJECTIVES

On completion of this chapter, the student should be able to:

- Describe the nature of hormonal imbalances in terms of hyposecretion and hypersecretion.
- Identify specific endocrine gland disorders.
- Describe the pathophysiologic bases and signs and symptoms of dysfunction of the endocrine glands.
- Describe factors influencing hormonal replacement therapies.
- Describe care of the patient undergoing surgery of specific endocrine glands.
- Specify learning needs of patients receiving hormonal replacement therapy.

PREREQUISITE READING

Long-Phipps, Chapter 29, pp. 941-990.

SELF-ASSESSMENT ACTIVITIES

I. Define the following terms.

Acromegaly
Addisonion crisis
Adrenal glands
Adrenocortiod-stimulating hormone (ACTH)
Androgen
Antidiuretic hormone (ADH)
Cortisol
Cushing's syndrome
Diabetes insipidus
Goiter
Graves' disease
Growth hormone (GH)
Hormones
Hyperthyroidism
Hypothyroidism
Oxytocin
Pituitary gland
Target cell
Tetany
Thyroid glands
Thyroid-stimulating hormone (TSH)
Thyroid storm

II. Answer the following questions.

1. List four endocrine glands.

2. List the pituitary hormones and their primary function.

Hormone **Function**

3. The adrenal cortex secretes two groups of hormones that are necessary for life. What are they? Give an example of each.

4. The adrenal medulla secretes which two important substances?

5. List five activities that increase intracranial pressure.

6. List five signs of addisonian crisis.

7. List the four signs of latent tetany.

III. Multiple choice

1. Which of the following is considered to be the master gland?
   a. Hypothalamus
   b. Adrenal
   c. Pituitary
   d. Thyroid
2. The way that hormones stimulate various responses in the body is a complex process. Primarily, they:
   a. Operate under genetic control
   b. Aim at specific target cells
   c. Travel to all parts of the body
   d. Stimulate all functions of the body
3. A distinguising feature of the endocrine system under which many hormones function is:
   a. The hypothalamus
   b. The thyroid gland
   c. Regulatory functions
   d. Feedback control
4. The adrenal medulla releases two types of catecholamines that have different effects in the body. Basically, these catecholamines:
   a. Maintain homeostasis
   b. Control all functioning
   c. Inhibit hormone control
   d. Control energy production
5. Serum cortisol levels, when measured, should be measured at:
   a. 8 AM
   b. Anytime during a 24-hour period
   c. 8 AM and 4 PM
   d. 4 PM and 12 AM
6. Which is a primary function of ACTH?
   a. Is responsible for secondary sex characteristics
   b. Stimulates thyroid gland to release T_3 and T_4
   c. Stimulates growth of all body cells, bones, and muscles
   d. Stimulates adrenal cortex to release glucocorticoids
7. Nancy Stewart has had a transsphenoidal adenomectomy. She is leaking CSF beneath the left nasal packing. Which nursing action would be most appropriate?
   a. Keep her flat in bed
   b. Suction the nasal cavity frequently
   c. Place her on bedrest in a Fowler's position
   d. Apply an ice collar to her neck

8. Absence of ADH may result in:
   a. Excessive output of dilute urine
   b. Decrease in urinary output
   c. Fluid volume excess
   d. Excess weight gain
9. Provocative testing is used for assessing pituitary function. The purpose of provocative testing is to:
   a. Inhibit the release of a particular hormone
   b. Stimulate release of a particular hormone
   c. Stimulate the buildup of products in the target organs that the hormone stimulates
   d. Stimulate the buildup of metabolic end-products
10. The most prominent findings in Addison's disease are:
   a. Hypotension and hypoglycemia
   b. Hypertension and headaches
   c. Sodium and fluid deficits
   d. Hypokalemia and edema
11. Following an adrenalectomy, the patient should be monitored very closely because:
   a. Severe fluctuations in hormone balance
   b. Increased intracranial pressure commonly occurs
   c. Paralysis of the lower extremities may occur
   d. Patients are high-risk for infections
12. Endemic goiters can be prevented by:
   a. Encouraging use of iodized salt
   b. Restricting the intake of caffeine
   c. Encouraging intake of calcium supplements with vitamin D
   d. Avoiding the use of harsh mouthwashes
13. A major nursing concern in caring for the patient with hyperthyroidism is:
   a. Providing adequate rest
   b. Keeping the patient warm
   c. Preventing weight gain
   d. Controlling edema

IV. Write a teaching plan for a patient requiring cortisol replacement.

SUGGESTED READINGS

Donham, J: The weakness of steroids, Am J Nurs 86:917-919, Aug 1986.
Describes manifestations of steroid myopathy, why it occurs, laboratory findings, and nursing assessments and interventions for steroid myopathy.

Hahn, AB, and others: Endocrine hormones and drugs affecting the endocrine system. In Mosby's Pharmacology in nursing, St Louis, 1986, The CV Mosby Co.

Larson, CA: The critical path of adrenocortical insufficiency, Nursing 14:66-69, Oct 1984.
Describes the prevention, cause, signs and symptoms, and management during crisis through use of a case study.

Propst, CL: Nursing care of a patient undergoing transsphenoidal hypophysectomy, J Neurosurg Nurs 15:332-338, Dec 1983.
Explains disorders that required use of this type of surgery, what to tell the patient, preoperative care, postoperative care and complications.

Chapter 30

The Patient with Hepatic, Biliary, and Pancreatic Problems

BRENDA GOODNER

CHAPTER OBJECTIVES

On completion of this chapter, the student should be able to:

- Describe preventive measures for hepatitis.
- Differentiate between focal and diffuse hepatocellular disorders, and explain the pathophysiologic basis for common manifestations of diffuse liver disorders.
- Differentiate between toxic and viral hepatitis, acute and chronic hepatitis, and among hepatitis A, B, D, and non-A, non-B.
- Explain the pathophysiologic bases for the symptoms of cirrhosis.
- Describe care of the patient with a diffuse liver disorder including control of gastrointestinal bleeding.
- Describe the nature of cholecystitis, cholelithiasis, and cancer of the biliary system, types of surgery, and care of the patient experiencing biliary surgery.
- Explain the pathophysiologic bases for signs and symptoms of pancreatitis and pancreatic tumors, and explain care of the patient during an acute phase and following surgery.
- Develop patient outcomes and nursing plans for patients exhibiting common signs and symptoms of hepatic dysfunction.

PREREQUISITE READING

Long-Phipps, Chapter 30, pp. 991-1044.

SELF-ASSESSMENT ACTIVITIES

I. Define the following terms.

Albumin	Cholelithiasis	Jaundice
Ascites	Cirrhosis	Pancreas
Biliary system	Encephalopathy	Pancreatitis
Bilirubin	Glycogenesis	Paracentesis
Blakemore-Sengstaken tube	Glyconeogenesis	T tube
Cholecystectomy	Hepatic system	
Cholecystitis	Hepatitis	

II. Answer the following questions.

1. List the five major liver functions.

2. Name the five signs and symptoms of peritonitis.

3. Describe the correct technique in examination and percussion of the liver.

4. List eight nursing interventions when a liver biopsy is taken.

5. What are six signs and symptoms of cholecystitis?

6. What are seven signs and symptoms of a patient suffering a relapse of pancreatitis?

III. List the following characteristics of hepatitis.

	Hepatitis A	**Hepatitis B**	**Non-A, non-B**
Transmission			
Incubation period			
Secretions that have been found to contain infective agent			
Clinical onset			
High-risk groups			

IV. Multiple choice

1. The process by which the liver forms new glucose from amino acids and lactic acids is:
   - **a.** Glycogenolysis
   - **b.** Gluconeogenesis
   - **c.** Protein metabolism
   - **d.** Protein catabolism
2. Bile production is one of the major functions of the liver. Where is bile stored?
   - **a.** Liver
   - **b.** Pancreas
   - **c.** Gallbladder
   - **d.** Stomach
3. The patient with hepatitis A must be placed on:
   - **a.** Respiratory isolation
   - **b.** Enteric isolation
   - **c.** Blood/body fluid precautions
   - **d.** Protective isolation
4. The source of hepatitis A is:
   - **a.** Primarily person-to-person through fecal contamination or contaminated food and water
   - **b.** Primarily from sexual contact with an infected person who does not show symptoms of the disease
   - **c.** Primarily contaminated needles from a person who has some form of hepatitis
   - **d.** Primarily through blood transfusions of improperly prepared blood
5. What kind of isolation is required for the patient with hepatitis B and non-A, non-B hepatitis?
   - **a.** Enteric
   - **b.** Respiratory
   - **c.** Strict
   - **d.** Blood/body fluids
6. Delta hepatitis can occur only if:
   - **a.** The victim comes in contact with infective blood
   - **b.** Sexual contact is made with infective person
   - **c.** Hepatitis A virus is present
   - **d.** Hepatitis B virus is present

Mr. Jonas is taken to the emergency room after being involved in an automobile accident. He was the driver of the car and suffered trauma to the liver when he hit the steering wheel.

7. The major emergency complication Mr. Jonas is most likely to suffer is:
   - **a.** Cardiac arrest
   - **b.** Hepatic arrest
   - **c.** Hypovolemic shock
   - **d.** Vasogenic shock
8. Another major complication of liver trauma is peritonitis. This occurs when:
   - **a.** The liver becomes infected after trauma
   - **b.** Bile and blood leak into the abdominal cavity
   - **c.** Blood supply to the liver is shut off
   - **d.** Surrounding organs of biliary system become infected
9. Why is hypovolemic shock such a major complication of liver trauma?
   - **a.** The liver has little blood supply
   - **b.** The liver has only two major vessels
   - **c.** The liver receives only unoxygenated blood
   - **d.** The liver is a highly vascular organ
10. Cirrhosis develops with several vague signs and symptoms over a long period of time. In the more advanced stage, signs and symptoms are:
    - **a.** Anorexia and constipation
    - **b.** Weight loss and indigestion
    - **c.** Pain and malnutrition
    - **d.** Jaundice and ascites
11. Nutrition is a major focus of nursing care of the cirrhosis patient. The restrictions for meal planning will include:
    - **a.** Sodium and fluids
    - **b.** Fats and protein
    - **c.** Sodium and seasonings
    - **d.** Protein and carbohydrates

12. There are three types of cirrhosis of the liver and many probable causes. The most common type in the United States is called portal cirrhosis. The exact cause is unknown. However, the most common predisposing factors are:
    a. Smoking and malnutrition
    b. Smoking and alcoholism
    c. Alcoholism and malnutrition
    d. Heredity and alcoholism
13. Portal hypertension can develop from the damage caused by cirrhosis. The most common and most dangerous complication of portal hypertension is:
    a. Ascites
    b. Cardiac arrest
    c. Hepatic coma
    d. Esophageal varices
14. In addition to pain, what other discomfort will the nurse assess in a patient with hepatic dysfunction?
    a. Palpitations
    b. Dizziness
    c. Pruritus
    d. Diaphoresis
15. In palpating the liver, it is abnormal if:
    a. It is palpable at all
    b. It is felt more than 1 cm below costal margins
    c. More than half of the size is palpable
    d. The whole liver is not easily palpable
16. After liver biopsy, the best position for the patient is:
    a. High-Fowler's
    b. Prone
    c. Supine
    d. Right lateral
17. A patient is scheduled for a liver biopsy. In preparing the patient for this test you should:
    a. Explain that the patient will be NPO for 24 hours before the exam
    b. Practice with the patient so he or she will be able to hold his or her breath for 1 minute
    c. Explain that the patient will be receiving a laxative to prevent a distended bowel from applying pressure on the liver
    d. Explain that the patient will be on bed rest for 24 hours after the test
18. The intervention of choice for most patients with cholelithiasis or cholecystitis is:
    a. Antibiotics
    b. Surgery
    c. Low-fat diet
    d. Vitamin K
19. A patient with jaundice is scheduled for an oral cholecystogram. It is most important that you determine:
    a. Whether the patient has had this test before, since it should not be repeated
    b. Whether the patient can tolerate fat, since ingestion of a high-fat meal will be necessary
    c. The patient's prothrombin time, since there is a risk of bleeding
    d. The patient's allergy history, since the dye contains iodine

Mrs. Young is a 44-year-old woman admitted with jaundice. She has been well until 4 days before admission. Her only complaints are jaundice, being tired, being weaker than usual, and pruritus. She is admitted for tests to diagnose the cause of the jaundice. A variety of tests are scheduled to see if Mrs. Young has liver disease. One of the tests is for urine urobilinogen.

20. The test is:
    a. A 24-hour urine collection
    b. Collected in the morning
    c. Followed by special medication
    d. Drawn in conjunction with other tests
21. The patient with pancreatitis will most often complain of:
    a. Pain
    b. Nausea
    c. Distention
    d. Fever

V. Write a nursing care plan for the following.

1. A patient with cirrhosis.

2. The postoperative care of a patient undergoing liver surgery.

SUGGESTED READINGS

Nursing Grand Rounds: Managing intractable pain with methadone (case study), Nurs 85 15(5):32-37, 1985.
Panel discussion of analgesics, table comparing morphine and methadone.

Pagean, MG, and others: New analgesic therapy relieves cancer pain without oversedation, Nurs 85 15(4):48-49, 1985. Intraspinal route for administration of narcotics.

Peternel, E: A high-tech approach to a GI problem . . . endoscopic retrograde cholangiopancreatography—ERCP . . . gallstones, RN 48:44-47, June 1985.
Describes what ERCP involves, patient preparation, and what it is used for.

Smith, CE: Assessing the liver, Nursing 15:36-37, July 1985.
Describes techniques of palpation, percussion, and auscultation, related anatomy and physiology, and abnormal findings.

Chapter 31

The Patient with Gastrointestinal Problems

MARY S. NICHOLS

CHAPTER OBJECTIVES

On completion of this chapter, the student should be able to:

- Describe measures for prevention and early detection of gastrointestinal (GI) disorders.
- Describe the nature of and nursing interventions for common inflammatory disorders of the mouth (stomatitis), stomach (gastritis), intestines (enteritis), and appendix (appendicitis).
- Describe the causes of dysphagia and heartburn and related therapeutic interventions.
- Differentiate gastric and duodenal ulcers and describe therapeutic modalities and patient teaching for peptic ulcer.
- Explain malabsorption syndrome and nursing interventions.
- Differentiate ulcerative colitis, Crohn's disease, and diverticular disease, and the care required for each.
- Describe the nature and care of the patient with intestinal obstruction, including hernias.
- Describe therapeutic modalities for patients with cancer of the mouth, stomach, and bowel, especially surgery.
- Describe the care of the person with a stoma for fecal diversion.
- Differentiate anorectal lesions and postoperative nursing care for rectal surgery.

PREREQUISITE READING

Long-Phipps, Chapter 31, pp. 1045-1122.

SELF-ASSESSMENT ACTIVITIES

I. Define the following terms.

Achalasia
Aphthous stomatitis
Aphthous ulcer
Barium enema
Body mass index
Borborygmi
Cardiotomy
Celiac disease
Colonoscopy
Chyme
Defecation
Deglutition
Dental caries
Dysphagia
Endoscopy
Erythroplakia
Esophagogastrostomy
Fetor oris
Gastric analysis
Gastric bypass
Gastric partitioning
Gastritis
Gastropexy
Gastrostomy
Gingivae
Gingivitis
Hemiglossectomy
Herpes simplex
Hiatal hernia
Ileocecal valve
Intramural plexus
Kwashiorkor
Leukoplakia
Lymphopenia
Melena
Mucositis
Obesity
Obstipation
Orthodontist
Paralytic ileus
Parotitis
Peptic ulcer
Periapical abscess
Peristalsis
Plaque
Pyorrhea
Rugae
Sgimoidoscopy
Steatorrhea
Stomatitis
Stool guaiac
Tartar
Tonus contractions
Tropical sprue
Vagotomy
Villi
Xerostomia

II. Multiple choice

1. The process of digestion begins in the:
   a. Mouth
   b. Small intestine
   c. Stomach
   d. Large intestine
2. Which of the following structures prevents the reflux of stomach contents into the esophagus?
   a. Pyloric sphincter
   b. Cardiac sphincter
   c. Esophageal sphincter
   d. Mitral sphincter
3. Food is propelled through the stomach and intestines by:
   a. Gravity
   b. Peristalsis
   c. Decreasing the stimulation of the intramural plexus
   d. Rugae
4. Two substances that control digestive functioning of the stomach are:
   a. Amylase and ptyalin
   b. Chyme and pepsin

Sam Martin, age 59, has cancer of the mouth. The tongue and pharynx are affected.

5. Tumors of the oral cavity:
   a. Are largely basal cell type carcinomas
   b. Have a poor prognosis
   c. Are more common in women than men
   d. Have a higher cure rate than tumors of the lip
6. Tumors of the mouth are believed to be due to:
   a. Alcoholism and heavy smoking
   b. Excessive intake of hot, spicy foods
   c. Heredity and poor dental hygiene
   d. Malnutrition and excessive exposure to ultraviolet rays

Several months after completing chemotherapy, Sam is readmitted and placed in a private room after the radiologist inserts two radioactive needles in Sam's tongue.

7. Having radioactive needles implanted in the tongue predisposes Sam to all of the following problems *except*:
   a. Increased salivation and drooling
   b. Dryness of the mouth
   c. Inflammation of the mucous membranes
   d. Dental decay
8. The incidence of cancer of the esophagus is highest among:
   a. Persons who consume large amounts of caffeinated beverages
   b. Smokers and alcoholics
   c. Persons who consume a low-fiber diet
   d. Persons who frequently consume hot, spicy foods

Don Jacobs, age 36, is admitted to the hospital with a diagnosis of acute peptic ulcer disease. He states that he has been taking cimetidine (Tagamet) and Amphogel at home to keep the ulcer under control.

9. Antacids:
   a. Should be given 30 minutes before meals
   b. Are given to neutralize gastric acid
   c. In tablet form are more effective than those in liquid form
   d. Inhibit gastric secretions

10. A major problem Don would be prone to developing because of prolonged use of Amphogel is:
    a. Nausea
    b. Constipation
    c. Hypercalcemia
    d. Flatulence
11. Cimetidine (Tagamet) achieves its effect by:
    a. Neutralizing gastric acid
    b. Coating the lining of the stomach
    c. Blocking the histamine receptor
    d. Stimulating the secretion of gastrin
12. When he is ready for discharge, the nurse should instruct Don to:
    a. Use bicarbonate of soda when painful attacks occur
    b. Eat a bedtime snack that is high in protein and fat
    c. Take prescribed Amphogel along with prescribed cimetadine (Tagamet)
    d. Avoid smoking and the use of alcohol
13. Because of his peptic ulcer, Don is prone to all of the following complications *except*:
    a. Hemorrhage
    b. Perforation
    c. Obstruction
    d. Epigastric pain
14. To determine whether Don is experiencing GI bleeding, the nurse would look for all of the following *except*:
    a. Positive stool guiac
    b. Hematemesis
    c. Epistaxis
    d. Black tarry stool
15. The nurse assesses Don frequently for manifestations of perforation. Which of the following is not a manifestation of perforation?
    a. Severe, sharp abdominal pain
    b. Rapid pulse and respirations
    c. Diaphoresis
    d. Epigastric fullness
16. Don's ulcer perforates. The nurse notifies the physician immediately. Emergency surgery is planned. Which of the following positions is most appropriate for Don while awaiting transportation to the O.R.?
    a. Low Fowler's
    b. Supine
    c. Prone
    d. Sim's
17. Stress ulcers:
    a. Are caused by excessive emotional stress
    b. Are manifested by diarrhea and steatorrhea
    c. Can lead to the same complications associated with peptic ulcer disease
    d. Are caused by a tumor of the pancreas
18. Which diagnostic test confirms a diagnosis of cancer of the stomach?
    a. Endoscopy with biopsy
    b. Upper GI series
    c. CEA (carcinoembryonic antigen) test
    d. Gastric analysis
19. The primary treatment for cancer of the stomach is:
    a. Use of antacids and histamine receptor blockers
    b. Gastrectomy
    c. Chemotherapy
    d. Radiation therapy

20. When a patient returns to the nursing unit after a gastroscopy, the nurse should:
  a. Keep the patient NPO until the gag reflex returns
  b. Instruct the patient to remain in bed for at least 4 hours
  c. Encourage oral intake of warm liquids
  d. Assess the patient for possible bowel incontinence

21. Preparation of the patient for a colonoscopy would involve all of the following *except:*
  a. Administration of a laxative or enema the day before the procedure
  b. Obtaining written consent from the patient
  c. Informing the patient that x-ray films will be taken after the dye has been injected into the rectum
  d. Keeping the patient NPO after midnight on the evening before the procedure

22. Patients who have had a subtotal gastrectomy (Bilroth I) often experience the dumping syndrome. The dumping syndrome is caused by:
  a. Rapid entry of hyperosmolar chyme directly into the jejunum
  b. Rapid entry of hyposmolar chyme directly into the jejunum
  c. Rapid entry of hyperosmolar chyme directly into the ileum
  d. Rapid entry of isotonic chyme directly into the duodenum

23. Clinical manifestations of the dumping syndrome include all of the following *except:*
  a. Diaphoresis
  b. Palpitations
  c. Faintness
  d. Hunger

24. To prevent the dumping syndrome, patients should be advised to:
  a. Eat a high-carbohydrate, low-fat, high-protein diet
  b. Take an antacid before each meal
  c. Avoid taking fluids with meals
  d. Exercise immediately after eating

25. Nursing care of the patient who has had a total gastrectomy (esophagojejunostomy) would involve all of the following *except:*
  a. Providing instructions about lifetime replacement therapy of vitamin B_{12}
  b. Anticipating the need for frequent emptying of the bottle collecting the nasogastric (N/G) tube drainage
  c. Observing the patient for manifestations of malabsorption
  d. Providing wound care to the thoracic incision

26. Following gastric surgery, patients always have a nasogastric tube in place. The nasogastric tube is removed when:
  a. Peristalsis return
  b. The patient begins to complain of hunger
  c. The patient no longer experiences severe abdominal pain
  d. The wound closure device (staples, sutures) are removed

27. Following a barium enema or upper GI series the most important nursing goal would be to:
  a. Prevent constipation
  b. Prevent fecal incontinence
  c. Maintain adequate nutritional intake
  d. Restore normal urinary elimination

28. Which of the following provides the most accurate way of confirming correct placement of a nasogastric tube?
  a. Aspirating gastric content
  b. Instilling air into the tube and listening for a roar over the epigastric area
  c. Seeing no bubbling when the end of the tube is placed in water
  d. Instilling a small amount of water into the tube and listening for a gurgling sound over the epigastric area

29. To facilitate passage of the Miller-Abbott tube into the small intestine, the nurse should do all of the following *except:*
  a. Encourage ambulation
  b. Reposition the patient every 2 hours
  c. Advance the tube to a prescribed distance at prescribed intervals
  d. Give the patient water to drink at regular intervals

30. Metabolic acidosis is a primary imbalance that can occur with prolonged:
  a. Intestinal suctioning
  b. Gastric suctioning

31. The most prominent manifestation of malabsorption of fats is:
  a. Steatorrhea
  b. Fatigue
  c. Increased flatulence
  d. Constipation

32. Individuals with a lactase deficiency have an intolerance to:
  a. Wheat
  b. Eggs
  c. Milk and milk products
  d. Simple sugars

33. When patients with a lactase deficiency consume foods that contain lactose, they will experience all of the following *except:*
  a. Abdominal distention
  b. Constipation
  c. Diarrhea
  d. Increased flatulence

34. Persons with celiac disease:
  a. Should avoid foods that contain wheat, rye, barley, and oats
  b. Should avoid tea, beer, and carbonated beverages
  c. Should avoid corn and soybean flour
  d. No longer have to adhere to dietary restrictions after adolescence

35. The major problem that results from paralytic ileus is:
  a. Obstruction
  b. Hemorrhage
  c. Peritonitis
  d. Perforation

36. Which of the following would not be characteristic of paralytic ileus?
  a. Vomiting
  b. Diarrhea
  c. Absent bowel sounds
  d. Abdominal distention

37. Which of the following would be used to decompress the stomach when paralytic ileus occurs?
  a. Laxatives
  b. Miller-Abbott tube connected to suction
  c. Salem sump tube connected to suction
  d. Manually applying pressure to the abdomen

III. Match each term below with the appropriate definition.

a. Achalasia
b. Dysphagia
c. Mucositis
d. Aphthous stomatitis
e. Gingivitis
f. Gastric partitioning
g. Cardiotomy
h. Kwashiorkor

1. ______ Canker sore
2. ______ Severe protein-calorie malnutrition
3. ______ Absence of peristalsis in the esophagus
4. ______ Difficulty swallowing
5. ______ Surgical intervention for obesity
6. ______ Inflammation of the mucous membranes
7. ______ Inflammation of the gums
8. ______ Widening of the esophagus at its junction with the stomach

IV. Match the type of stool commonly associated with the physiologic conditions listed below.

a. Cancer of the colon
b. Partial obstruction of descending colon
c. Parasitic infestations
d. Bleeding from the GI tract

1. ______ Black, tarry stools
2. ______ Diarrhea containing pus, mucous, and possible undigested food
3. ______ Alternating constipation and diarrhea
4. ______ Small, ribbon-shaped stools

5. List the three divisions of the small intestines.

6. List the three divisions of the large intestines.

V. Complete the chart below on ulcerative colitis, Crohn's disease, and irritable bowel syndrome.

	Ulcerative colitis	**Crohn's disease**	**Irritable bowel syndrome**
Area of involvement			
Extent of involvement			
Appearance of mucosa			
Cancer potential			
Character of stool			
Major complications			
Potential for cure			

VI. Write the answer to each of the following questions in the space provided.

1. What is the most prominent clinical manifestation of a hernia?

2. What is the best treatment for a hernia?

3. What discharge instructions should be given to the patient who has had a herniorrhaphy?

4. Why is a colon resection done for familiar polyposis?

5. What interventions are used to cleanse the bowel in preparation for colon surgery?

6. What type of diet should be followed to prevent diverticulosis?

7. Why should patients with an ileostomy *not* be given solid forms (tablets, capsules) of oral medications?

8. What dietary changes must the patient with an ileostomy follow?

9. What dietary changes must a patient with a colostomy follow?

10. What is the purpose of colostomy irrigations?

11. If a patient who has had a colostomy or ileostomy shows no fecal output on the first postoperative day, what should the nurse do? Why?

12. What type of drainage should the patient have from the ostomies below?

	Colostomy	Ileostomy
When functioning begins		
At 1 month		
At 1 year		

13. List at least four major complications associated with a fecal diversion ostomy.

14. Write a description of a normal stoma initially after surgery.

15. Can a female of childbearing age who has had a permanent colostomy as a result of ulcerative colitis conceive children?

VII. Match each term below with its appropriate definition.

a. Fecal impaction
b. McBurney's point
c. Meckel's diverticulum
d. Volvulus
e. Intussusception
f. Diverticulosis
g. Hernia
h. Hemorrhoids
i. Obstipation

1. _____ A twisting of the bowel
2. _____ The protrusion of an organ from its normal cavity through a defect
3. _____ An outpouching of the mucosal walls of the colon
4. _____ Varicose veins of the rectum
5. _____ An outpouching of the mucosal walls of the ileum
6. _____ Extremely hard stool that cannot be expelled
7. _____ Located midway between the umbilicus and the anterior right iliac crest
8. _____ A telescoping of a segment of the bowel onto itself
9. _____ Constipation

VIII. Select the best answer for each item.

1. Constipation can occur:
   - **a.** From any condition that leads to decreased absorption of water from the colon
   - **b.** By ignoring the urge to defecate
   - **c.** From any condition that is characterized by increased intestinal motility
   - **d.** From prolonged intake of a high-fiber diet
2. To prevent constipation, individuals should be instructed to do all *except:*
   - **a.** Eat a high-fiber diet
   - **b.** Drink 6 to 8 glasses of water daily
   - **c.** Engage in a daily exercise program
   - **d.** Use laxatives every other day
3. The definition of diarrhea is based upon:
   - **a.** The number of stools a patient has daily
   - **b.** The expulsion of a watery stool
   - **c.** The color of the stool
   - **d.** The appearance of undigested food particles in the stool
4. Care of the patient with diarrhea would include all *except:*
   - **a.** Avoiding caffeinated beverages
   - **b.** Encouraging small frequent feedings
   - **c.** Encouraging a high-fiber, high-protein diet
   - **d.** Assessing for fluid and electrolyte imbalances
5. On the second postoperative day, a patient who had abdominal surgery complains of severe abdominal discomfort caused by flatulence. The best action for the nurse to take to relieve flatulence would be to:
   - **a.** Ambulate the patient more frequently
   - **b.** Apply a hot water bottle to the patient's abdomen
   - **c.** Advise the patient to maintain a supine position while in bed
   - **d.** Administer the prescribed analgesic
6. A bowel-training program should:
   - **a.** Be based on the patient's pattern of defecation
   - **b.** Include use of a low-fiber diet
   - **c.** Include restriction of liquid intake to 1000 ml/day
   - **d.** Involve daily use of enemas to regulate the bowels

Janice Carnes, age 25, is admitted to the clinical unit with a diagnosis of probable appendicitis.

7. On assessing Janice, the nurse would anticipate finding all of the following *except:*
   - **a.** Elevated temperature
   - **b.** Low WBC (white blood count)
   - **c.** Severe abdominal pain in the right lower quadrant
   - **d.** Severe abdominal pain in the epigastric area
8. Stat lab work has been done. While awaiting the results of the tests, care for Janice would include:
   - **a.** Administering medication for pain
   - **b.** Applying a warm, dry compress to her abdomen
   - **c.** Providing sips of warm liquids
   - **d.** Maintaining bed rest
9. The major complication associated with appendicitis is:
   - **a.** Perforation with resultant peritonitis
   - **b.** Hemorrhage with resultant shock
   - **c.** Bowel obstruction with resultant gangrene
   - **d.** Renal failure with resultant heart failure
10. Manifestations of peritonitis include all *except:*
    - **a.** Severe abdominal pain
    - **b.** Rigid, boardlike abdomen
    - **c.** Soft, boggy abdomen
    - **d.** Decreasing blood pressure, increasing pulse, and respiration

11. Inflammatory bowel disease:
  a. Is found more frequently in rural areas
  b. Is hereditary
  c. Has an unknown cause
  d. Is caused by an infectious process

12. Which diagnostic test is most helpful in distinguishing ulcerative colitis from Crohn's disease?
  a. Endoscopy
  b. Stool for occult blood
  c. Barium enema
  d. Upper GI series

13. Sulfasalazine (Azulfidine) is the drug of choice for treating:
  a. Parasitic infections
  b. Irritable bowel syndrome
  c. Crohn's disease
  d. Cancer of the colon

14. What type of fecal diversion stoma is advocated for surgical management of Crohn's disease?
  a. Ileostomy
  b. Colostomy
  c. Ileoconduit
  d. Gastrostomy

15. Patients with ulcerative colitis should be advised to:
  a. Drink plenty of milk
  b. Eat lots of raw fruits and vegetables
  c. Reduce the intake of fluids
  d. Avoid alcohol and caffeinated beverages

16. Anal fissure, anal abscess, and anal fistula are related disorders in that:
  a. All three can lead to hemorrhoid formation
  b. All three can best be prevented with daily use of a high-fiber diet
  c. All three can lead to diverticula disease
  d. Anal fissure can lead to abscess, which can lead to fistula

17. To provide comfort for the patient who has had surgery for an anorectal lesion (fistula, fissure, or abscess), the nurse will do all of the following *except:*
  a. Administer a stool softener daily
  b. Administer sitz baths
  c. Provide a foam pad to sit on
  d. Apply an analgesic ointment to the anal area

18. To prevent stricture of the anorectal area post-hemorrhoidectomy, the nurse would:
  a. Give a sitz bath twice daily
  b. Administer stool softeners daily
  c. Insert a rectal packing
  d. Insert a rectal tube

19. Signs and symptoms of bowel obstruction include all of the following *except:*
  a. Obstipation
  b. Absence of bowel sounds
  c. Abdominal distention
  d. Low-pitched bowel sounds

20. The best method of evaluating the extent of abdominal distention is to:
  a. Weigh the patient daily
  b. Auscultate for bowel sounds more frequently
  c. Measure the patient's abdominal girth daily
  d. Percuss the abdomen more frequently

21. Which type of hernia does not involve a protrusion of a loop of intestine?
    a. Direct inguinal
    b. Indirect inguinal
    c. Hiatal
    d. Umbilical
22. Which of the following preoperative activities would be most important for the patient undergoing closure of a colostomy?
    a. Bowel cleansing
    b. Teaching how to splint when coughing
    c. Teaching muscle-strengthening exercises
    d. Practicing good use of body mechanics
23. What type of fecal diversion stoma will be created with an abdominoperineal resection?
    a. Ileostomy
    b. Permanent colostomy
    c. Ileoconduit
    d. Temporary colostomy
24. Constipation is a major problem that may occur with which type of fecal diversion stoma?
    a. Colostomy
    b. Ileostomy
    c. Both

IX. Complete the chart below on parasitic infections.

	Amebiasis	**Trichinosis**
Species of parasite		
Mode of transmission		
Diagnostic test		
Method(s) of prevention		
Treatment		
Site(s) where parasite ultimately settles in the host		

CASE STUDY

Steve Provost, age 58, is admitted to the hospital for diagnostic tests. He states that for the past 4 months his appetite has been poor and that he feels tired all the time. He also states that he has lost 35 lb and that he has an upset stomach most of the time. A gastroscopy with biopsy is performed. The results revealed cancer of the stomach. A total body scan is performed to assess the extent of metastasis.

A partial gastrectomy (Bilroth I) is performed. Postoperatively, Mr. Provost returns to the unit with the following orders:

N/G to low-intermittent suction
1000 ml D-5-Normosol-M at 125 ml/hr
Foley catheter to drainage bag
Intake and output every 8 hours
NPO
Change abdominal dressing prn
Demerol 50-100 mg, IM every 4 hours prn for pain
Irrigate N/G with normal saline prn

When the nurse enters Mr. Provost's room to obtain his vital signs, he begins to cry and states, "I've lived a good life. I know now that it's just a matter of time."

A. Answer the following questions in the space provided.

1. What would the nurse have to do to prepare Mr. Provost for the gastroscopy?

2. What nursing care would Mr. Provost require after the gastroscopy?

3. What must the nurse do to ensure an accurate assessment of N/G output when irrigating the N/G tube?

4. What would be the appropriate response for the nurse to make to Mr. Provost's tearful statement?

B. Complete the postgastrectomy care plan for Mr. Provost based on the assessment that has been documented.

Assessment	Planning	Interventions	Evaluation (assume that goal is met)
N/G connected to low intermittent suction and draining greenish fluid	*Nursing diagnosis:* Potential for complications related to (r/t) N/G suction. *Goal:* Experience no complications of N/G suctioning	1. 2. 3. 4. 5. 6.	1. No signs of electrolyte, fluid, or acid-base imbalance 2. 3.

Continued

Assessment	Planning	Interventions	Evaluation (assume that goal is met)
Complaining of incisional pain. This is patient's first postgastrectomy day. Last pain medication given 4 hours ago.	*Nursing diagnosis:* *Goal:*	1. Assist to position of comfort. Keep in low-Fowler's. If lying on back, raise knee gatch on bed slightly to relieve strain on abdominal muscles. 2.	1.
OR record reveals that 2 Penrose drains are in place beneath the dressing. Abdominal dressing has moderate amount of serosanguineous drainage.	*Nursing diagnosis:* *Goal:*	1. 2.	1. Skin beneath tape red and tender from frequent changing of tape during dressing changes; will apply Montgomery straps 2.

CLINICAL ACTIVITIES

1. If an enterostomal therapist is available in your community or agency, accompany him or her on rounds.
2. Explore your community to find out what agencies or organizations are available to help the ostomy patient adapt to their new body image and ostomy care.

SUGGESTED READINGS

Assess your care of the patient with peptic ulcer disease, Nurs 88 18(4):32U-32W, 1988.
Twenty-one multiple-choice items for reviewing this disease. Explanations of answers included.

Patras, AZ, and others: Gastrointestinal assessment: identifying significant problems, AORN J 40:726-731, Nov 1984.
Includes a detailed description of postoperative assessment of the gastrointestinal system. Major complications affecting the GI tract are described. A detailed case study is given of a patient with inflammatory bowel disease who undergoes a colon resection and appendectomy.

Patras, A, and others: Managing GI bleeding: it takes a two-track mind, Nurs 88 18(4), 1988.
Case study approach lists key history questions for the GI bleedings, including graphic illustrations, treatment, estimation of blood loss from surgical procedures, comfort measures, and discharge teaching.

Chapter 32

The Patient with Urinary Problems

MARY S. NICHOLS

CHAPTER OBJECTIVES

On completion of this chapter, the student should be able to:

- Describe interventions for urinary retention and urinary incontinence.
- Describe the causes and methods of prevention of urinary tract infections (UTIs). Differentiate between upper and lower UTI.
- Describe pathophysiologic differences among, signs and symptoms of, and therapeutic modalities and nursing interventions for glomerular disorders.
- Describe the pathophysiology of obstructive urinary disorders.
- Describe the pathophysiology and interventions for renal calculi.
- Compare different approaches to prostatectomy and describe the related nursing interventions.
- Describe the care of the person undergoing surgery of the urinary tract.
- Differentiate between acute and chronic renal failure, including pathophysiology, sign and symptoms, medical therapy, and nursing interventions.
- Explain the physiologic principles of dialysis and describe the types of dialysis and related care.
- Describe the care of the person with a kidney transplant.

PREREQUISITE READING

Long-Phipps, Chapter 32, pp.1123-1216.

SELF-ASSESSMENT ACTIVITIES

I. Define the following terms.

Acute tubular necrosis
Angiotensinogen
Anuria
Azotemia
BPH
Bruit
CAPD
Cystectomy
Cystitis
Cystometrogram
Cystoscopy
Dialysis
Diffusion
Dwell time
Dysuria
Epispadias
Erythropoietin
Frequency
Glomerular filtration rate (GFR)
Glomerulonephritis

Hematuria
Hemodialysis
Hesitancy
Homeostasis
Hydronephrosis
Hydroureter
Hypospadias
Intravenous pyelography
Litholapaxy
Lithotripsy
Nephrectomy
Nephrolithiasis
Nephron
Nephroplexy
Nephroptosis
Nephrosclerosis
Nephrostomy
Nephrotic syndrome
Nocturia
Oliguria
Osmosis

Osteodystrophy
Peritoneal dialysis
Polycystic disease
Polyuria
Pulsus paradoxus
Pyelolithotomy
Pyelonephritis
Renal colic
Renal insufficiency
Renin
Residual urine
Thrill
Trigone
TURP
Ultrafiltration
Uremia
Ureterolithotomy
Urethritis
Ureterostomy
Urinary incontinence
Urolithiasis

II. Identification

1. Label the kidney components in the illustration below.
2. Number the structures below according to the order of their involvement in the process by which urine is formed.

a. ______ Descending loop of Henle
b. ______ Urethra
c. ______ Glomerular capillaries
d. ______ Distal convoluted tubule
e. ______ Afferent arteriole
f. ______ Bowman's capsule
g. ______ Ureters
h. ______ Loop of Henle
i. ______ Proximal convoluted tubule
j. ______ Collecting ducts
k. ______ Ascending loop of Henle
l. ______ Bladder

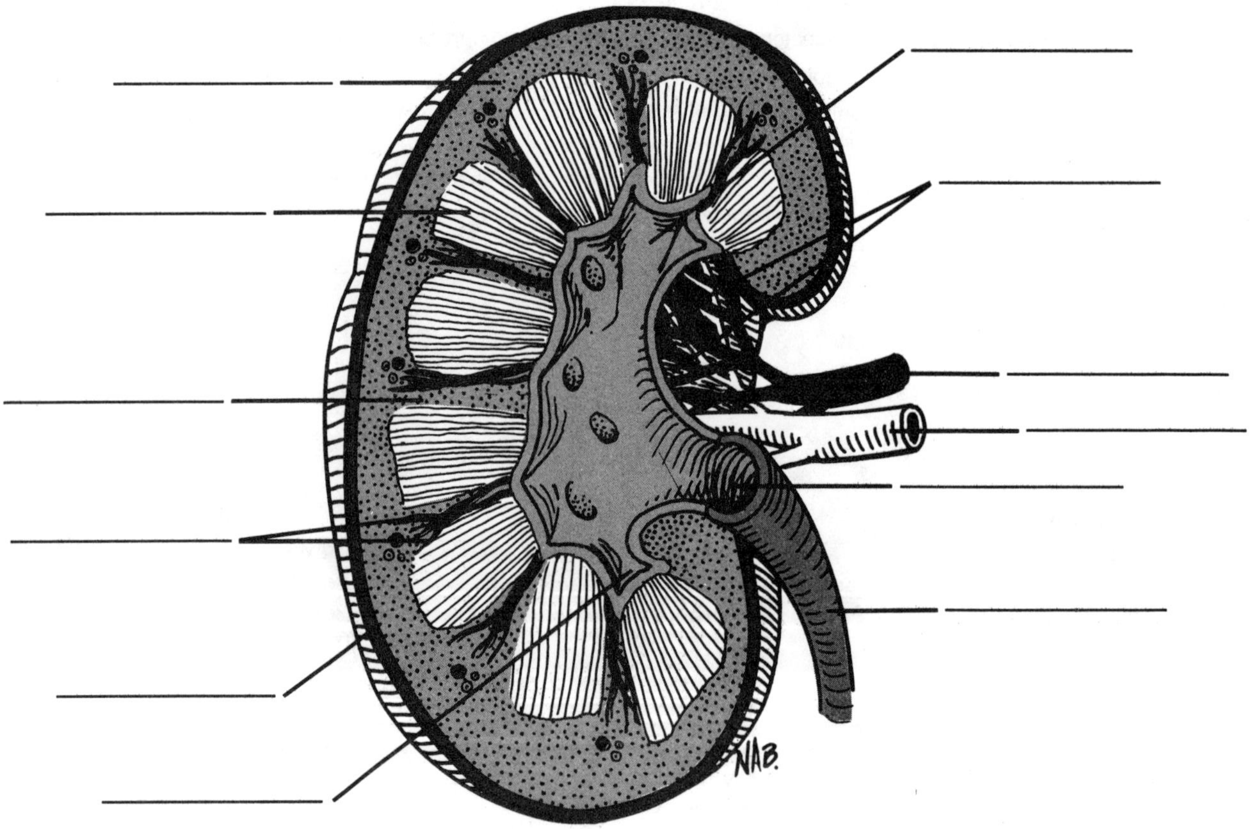

3. Label the parts of the urinary bladder and associated structures in the illustration below.

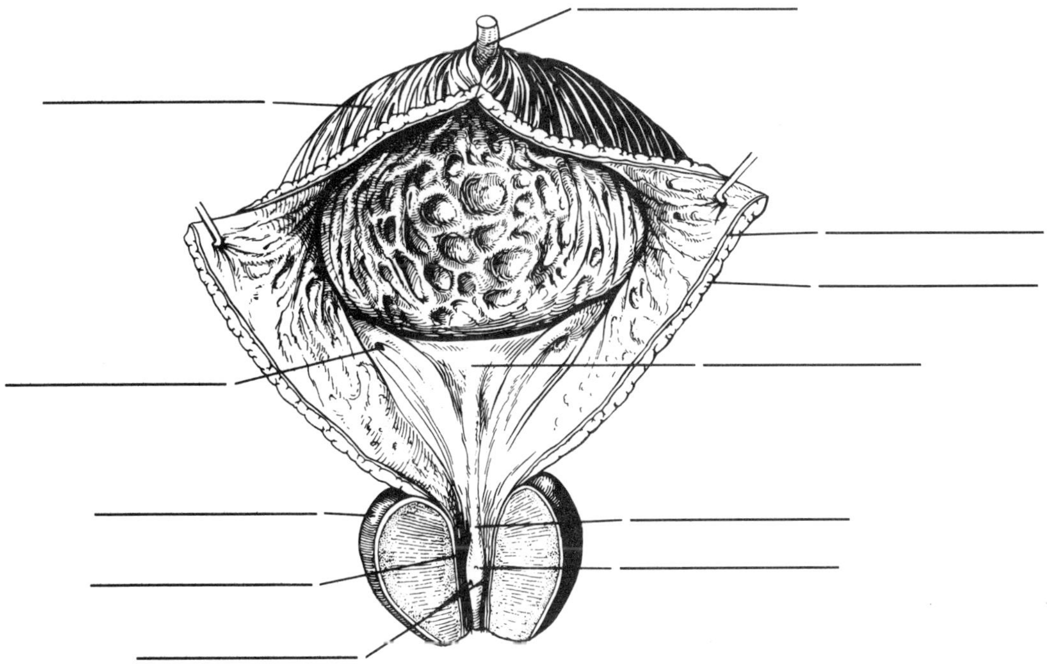

4. Identify the structures of the urinary tract in the illustration below.

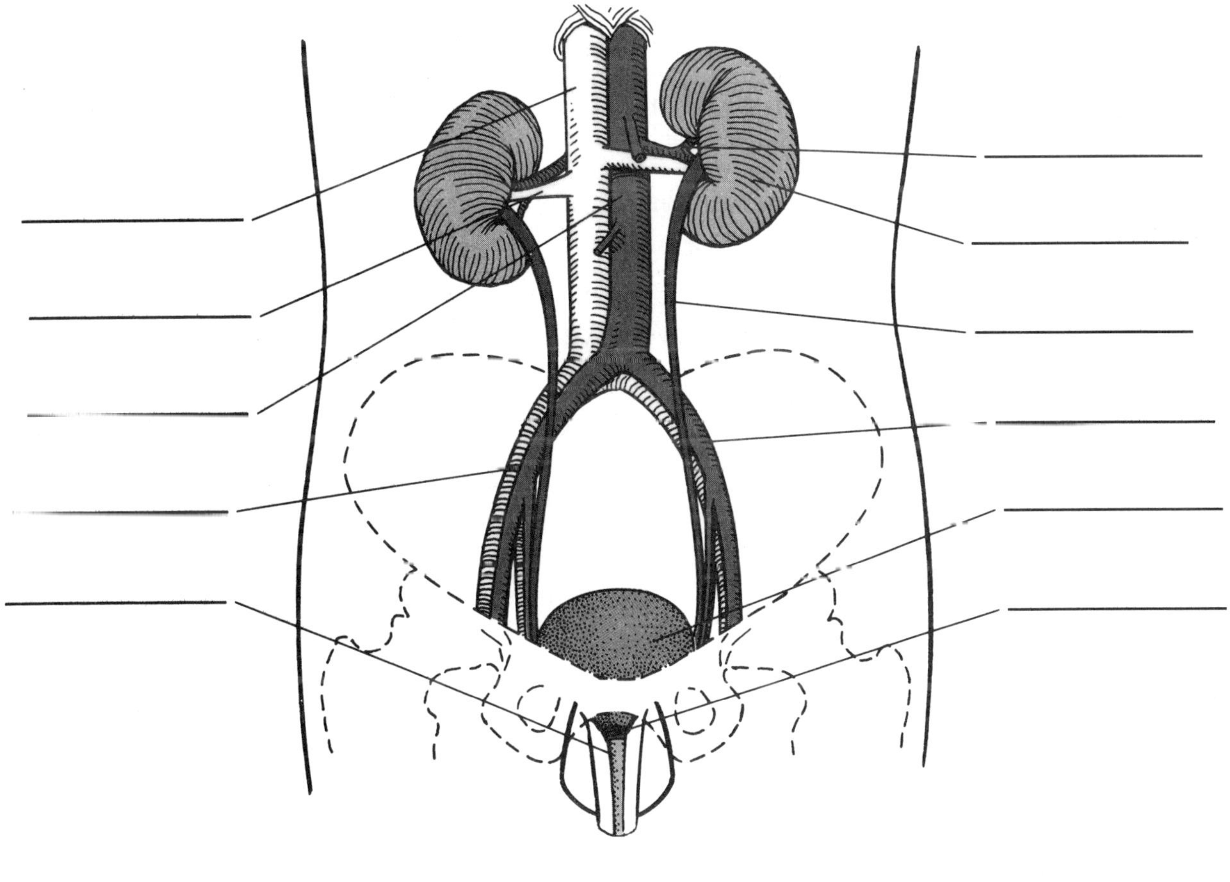

5. Label the nephron in the illustration below.

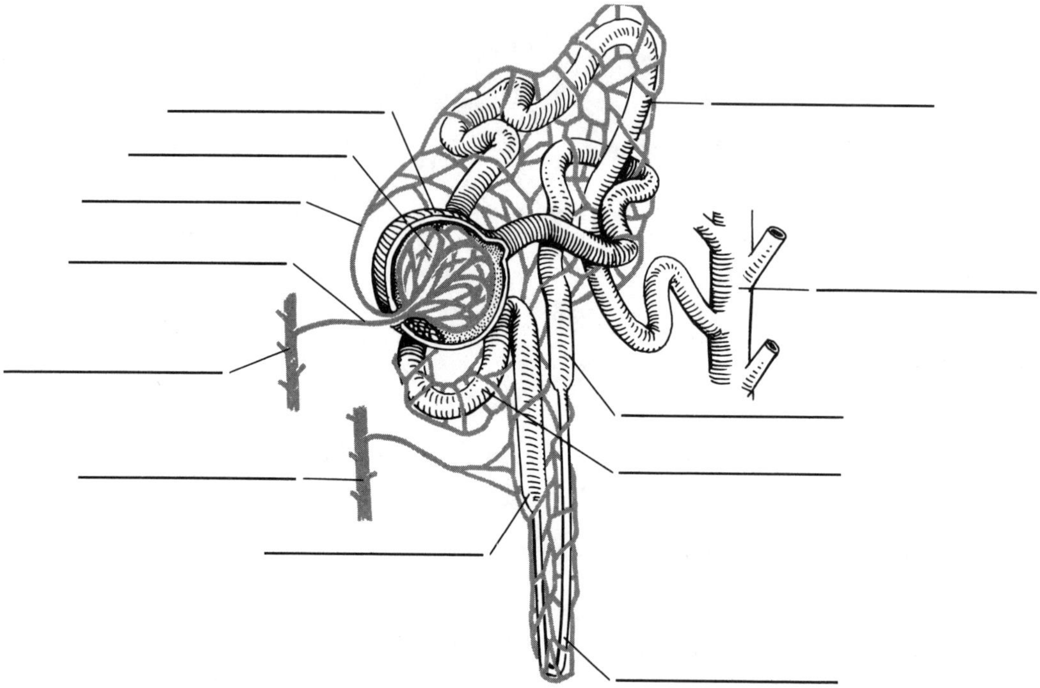

III. Circle the correct word in the description of the process of micturition.

The (detrusor/perineal) muscle within the wall of the bladder responds to increasing pressure within the bladder as it fills by (relaxing/contracting) to accommodate the volume. When the bladder fills to capacity, usually (50 to 100/150 to 350) ml of urine, the (sympathetic/parasympathetic) stretch receptors located within the bladder wall are (stimulated/suppressed). The impulses are transmitted through (afferent/efferent) fibers to the reflex arc for micturition. Impulses are then carried through the (afferent/efferent) fibers to the reflex arc to the bladder, causing (contraction/relaxation) of the detrusor muscle. The (internal/external) sphincter, which is normally closed, reciprocally opens and urine enters the posterior urethra. (Relaxation/Contraction) of the (internal/external) sphincter and perineal muscles follows and urine exits the body.

IV. Write your answers in the space provided.

1. Once an indwelling catheter is inserted and connected to a closed drainage system, what measures should a nurse use to maintain patency of the system and prevent UTI?

2. A comatose patient has a Foley catheter that is draining cloudy foul-smelling urine with large amounts of sediment. There is 120 ml of urine in the bedside bag. Acetic acid irrigations are ordered. You instill 60 ml of solution into the catheter manually. After removing the Asepto syringe to allow the solution to drain out, only 10 ml drains out. What would be appropriate actions to take? How will you calculate the patient's total urinary output?

3. What instructions would you give a patient with a Foley catheter about:
   a. Sexual intercourse

   b. Showers and tub baths

   c. Care of equipment at home

4. List three major problems that patients should be assessed for after a Foley catheter is removed.

5. Patients are taught to use a clean technique when performing intermittent self-catheterization at home, but when they are admitted to the hospital a sterile technique must be used. Why?

6. What effect does a cystectomy have on a patient's sexual functioning?

7. What are the major complications associated with urinary diversion procedures?

8. Why is preoperative bowel preparation necessary when a patient undergoes a cystectomy? What does bowel preparation consist of?

9. What are some factors that should be considered when planning a bladder retraining schedule for an incontinent patient?

10. Following removal of a Foley for a TURP, a male patient experiences incontinence. You plan to teach him perineal exercises. What instructions would you give him?

11. How would you instruct Mrs. L., a 38-year-old courtroom stenographer, to perform intermittent self-catheterization at home?

12. To what major class of antibiotics do kanamycin and gentamycin belong? What are the major toxic effects of this class of antibiotics? What should the nurse look for to determine toxicity?

13. What diagnostic test can be used to identify the source of chemical-induced nephritis?

14. What can be done to prevent chronic glomerulonephritis and nephrotic syndrome?

15. What is the primary cause of:

a. Renal artery stenosis

b. Nephrosclerosis

16. What is the first indication of diabetic nephropathy?

17. Why do nephrosclerosis, renal artery stenosis, and diabetic nephropathy ultimately lead to chronic renal failure?

18. What is the major factor that predisposes to renal calculi? Why? What is the most common type of renal calculi?

19. Which type of renal calculi precipitates in an acid urine? Which type precipitates in an alkaline urine?

20. Why is the prognosis poor for patients with tumors of the kidney?

21. Which type of prostatic surgery is associated with:

a. Leakage of urine onto the abdominal dressing?

b. Altered sexual functioning?

c. Incontinence?

V. **1.** Complete the drug chart below.

	Classification	**Action/use**	**Adverse reactions**	**Nursing considerations**
Propantheline (Probanthine)				
Bethanechol chloride (Urecholine)				

2. Complete the chart below. Underline the similarities between the two disorders.

	Pyelonephritis	Tuberculosis of the kidney
Mode of entry of organism		
Clinical findings		
How diagnosis is confirmed		

3. Complete the drug chart below.

Drugs	Action	Major side effects	Nursing considerations
Gantrisin			
Furadantin			
Pyridium			
Bactrim			
Pro-Banthine			
Thio-TEPA			
Zyloprim			
Kayexalate			
Sorbitol			
Prednisone			

4. Complete the chart below comparing acute glomerulonephritis with the nephrotic syndrome. In the column 'Primary clinical finding' list the findings from physical assessment of the patient and from diagnostic studies that correlate with the pathophysiological changes. See example given under acute glomerulonephritis.

	Acute glomerulonephritis	Primary clinical finding	Nephrotic syndrome	Primary clinical finding
Primary cause	Streptococcal infection from throat or skin	↑ ASO titer		
Primary pathologic changes				

5. A patient returns to the clinical unit following abdominal surgery. Eight hours have passed, and the patient has not voided. An intravenous infusion is running in her right hand at 100 cc/hr. You suspect that the patient is experiencing either suppression of the kidneys or retention. Under the appropriate headings, write the assessments you would make for each problem. See example given.

Urinary retention	**Kidney suppression**
Palpate bladder for distention	Check b/p for elevation, which indicates fluid overload

VI. Multiple choice

1. Mr. Carter is experiencing acute urinary retention secondary to enlargement of the prostate gland. Which intervention would be most appropriate to reestablish urine flow?
   a. Having him take a warm shower
   b. Administering bethanechol chloride (Urecholine)
   c. Having him stand upright and place hands in warm water
   d. Catheterizing him
2. Catheterization can be done for all of the following reasons *except:*
   a. To achieve continence
   b. To stimulate production of urine
   c. To permit irrigation of bladder
   d. To permit healing of urinary structures following surgery
3. All of the following measures are aimed at preventing UTI in patients with a Foley catheter *except:*
   a. Anchoring the tubing securely to the thigh
   b. Encouraging a fluid intake of at least 3 liters/day
   c. Cleansing the metal-catheter junction with soap and water twice daily
   d. Collecting urine specimens from the sample port using aseptic technique
4. The frequency of intermittent catheterization is determined by:
   a. The amount of urine the patient is able to void
   b. The size of catheter used
   c. The amount of residual urine
   d. The amount of fluid intake
5. Treatment of neurogenic bladder may include all *except:*
   a. Administration of bethanechol chloride (Urecholine)
   b. Use of the Crede method
   c. Cystectomy
   d. Intermittent catheterization

6. Mr. Kushner is a 72-year-old confused elderly patient. He is ambulatory and incontinent of urine. Which of the following interventions to control his incontinence would be *least* appropriate?
   - **a.** External condon catheter
   - **b.** Teaching perineal exercises
   - **c.** Bladder retraining
   - **d.** Disposable waterproof briefs
7. Mr. James has just returned to the clinical unit following a left nephrectomy. He is alert and oriented. Which assessment would be most important for the nurse to make next?
   - **a.** Bowel sounds
   - **b.** Skin integrity
   - **c.** Chest sounds
   - **d.** Urinary output
8. A patient has an ileal conduit. Urine is leaking around the pouch. The nurse decides to apply a new pouch. To prevent drainage of urine from the stoma onto the surrounding skin as it is being cleansed, the nurse should:
   - **a.** Have the patient plug the stoma opening with his finger
   - **b.** Use sterile technique when changing the pouch
   - **c.** Inset a rolled piece of gauze into the stoma opening
   - **d.** Have the patient stand over the commode
9. Urinary tract infections are more common in females than males because:
   - **a.** Females are more sexually active than males.
   - **b.** Females have a longer urethra than males.
   - **c.** The urethra of the female lies in close proximity to the rectum.
   - **d.** The male urethra has an s-shaped curve near the bladder, and the urethra of the female does not.
10. Nina Salomon, age 15, has UTI. She is placed on Bactrim q.i.d. To prevent recurrence of the infection, she should do all of the following *except*:
    - **a.** Drink 3 liters of fluids daily
    - **b.** Discontinue the Bactrim once symptoms are no longer present
    - **c.** Wipe perineum from front to back after toileting.
    - **d.** Return to doctor's office for repeat urine cultures after completion of drug therapy.
11. The most prominent clinical manifestation of UTI is:
    - **a.** Urgency and dysuria
    - **b.** Nocturia and incontinence
    - **c.** Hematuria and bladder spasms
    - **d.** Hesitancy and cloudy urine
12. Which of the following findings would be most significant for acute glomerulonephritis?
    - **a.** History of sore throat or impetigo
    - **b.** Painless hematuria
    - **c.** Flank pain and a palpable abdominal mass
    - **d.** Dysuria and urgency
13. Which drug would most likely be prescribed in the treatment of acute glomerulonephritis?
    - **a.** Furadantin
    - **b.** Gantrisin
    - **c.** Penicillin
    - **d.** Septra
14. For patients with acute glomerulonephritis, which intervention is aimed at reducing metabolic needs of the kidney so that healing can occur?
    - **a.** Restricting fluid intake
    - **b.** Administering antibiotics
    - **c.** A low-sodium diet
    - **d.** Bedrest
15. The primary pathology in chronic glumerulonephritis is:
    - **a.** Progressive sclerosis
    - **b.** Progressive formation of cysts
    - **c.** Malignant carcinoma
    - **d.** Progressive infection
16. Which of the following is not a clinical manifestation of the nephrotic syndrome?
    - **a.** Proteinuria
    - **b.** Hypolipidemia
    - **c.** Hypoalbuminemia
    - **d.** Generalized edema
17. Patients with the nephrotic syndrome may be placed on prednisone in order to:
    - **a.** Reduce protein loss
    - **b.** Prevent muscle wasting
    - **c.** Reduce inflammation
    - **d.** Stop hematuria

18. The most common organism causing pyelonephritis is:
    a. Escherichia coli
    b. Staphylococcus
    c. Streptococcus
    d. Clostridium
19. If a patient has recurring episodes of pyelonephritis, which diagnostic test would be used to assess the extent of structural damage to the kidney?
    a. CBC
    b. Urine culture
    c. Cystoscopy
    d. IVP
20. To remove by-products of inflammation and infection, patients with UTI should:
    a. Drink lots of fluids
    b. Take antibiotics as prescribed
    c. Be as active as possible
    d. Have a back massage to massage the kidneys
21. The most prominent clinical manifestation of renal artery stenosis is:
    a. Hematuria
    b. Flank pain
    c. Hypertension
    d. Proteinuria
22. Hydronephrosis is caused by:
    a. Accumulation of fluid in the peritoneal cavity
    b. An obstruction of the urinary tract
    c. Bacteria
    d. Fluid overload
23. Which condition does not contribute to the formation of calcium oxalate kidney stones?
    a. Immobilization
    b. Prolonged use of steroids
    c. Gout
    d. Hyperparathyroidism
24. Which type of renal calculi is caused by a genetic disorder of amino acid metabolism?
    a. Calcium oxalate
    b. Calcium phosphate
    c. Cystine
    d. Uric acid
25. With a TURP:
    a. There is a low midline abdominal incision through the bladder to the prostate gland
    b. There is no incision
    c. There is a small incision between the scrotum and rectum
    d. There is a low midline incision into the perineum
26. Following a TURP, a patient returns to the clinical unit with a 3-way Foley, which has a 30cc balloon, in place. The catheter is pulled very taut and taped securely to his thigh to apply traction. The purpose of applying traction on the catheter is to:
    a. Control bleeding
    b. Prevent deflation of the balloon
    c. Keep him from moving his leg
    d. Prevent bladder spasms
27. Which of the following discharge instructions would be inappropriate for the patient following a TURP?
    a. Avoid heavy lifting for at least 3 weeks.
    b. Use stool softeners or mild laxatives if needed.
    c. Drink at least 3 liters of fluids daily.
    d. You may resume sexual intercourse as soon as desired.
28. The most common sign of cancer of the urinary tract is:
    a. Flank pain
    b. Flank mass
    c. Unexplained weight loss
    d. Painless hematuria

Mr. Zanuck, a 44-year-old truck driver, suffered excessive blood loss from abdominal injuries he sustained when his truck overturned late one winter evening. When the ambulance brought him to the emergency room his blood pressure was 74/42, pulse was 124, and respirations were 26. A Foley catheter was inserted and 14 ml of dark concentrated urine was obtained. For the past 24 hours his urinary output has averaged 20 ml/hour. A diagnosis of acute renal failure is made. His wife tells the nurse that he routinely smokes about one-half pack of cigarettes daily and has at least two cans of beer after his dinner.

29. Which of the following contributed *most* to the development of acute renal failure in Mr. Zanuck?
    a. Age
    b. Occupation
    c. Excessive intake of beer
    d. Excessive blood loss
30. The severity of symptoms in acute renal failure depends on:
    a. The patient's previous health status
    b. The number of functioning nephrons
    c. The agent or substance causing renal failure
    d. The type of drugs used in the initial treatment of the disease
31. The physician orders an intravenous infusion of furosemide for Mr. Zanuck. Which of the following findings would indicate the desired therapeutic response of this drug?
    a. An increase in urinary output
    b. An increase in blood pressure
    c. A decrease in pulse rate
    d. A decrease in respiration
32. In spite of aggressive medical interventions, Mr. Zanuck remains oliguric. Since admission 24 hours ago, his intake has been 2500 cc and his urinary output 250 cc. Which of the following assessments would be most important for the nurse to make at this time?
    a. Palpate peripheral pulses
    b. Observe skin color
    c. Auscultate breath sounds
    d. Auscultate abdomen for peristalsis
33. The nurse checks the results of Mr. Zanuck's serum laboratory tests. The nurse would anticipate finding all of the following biochemical imbalances *except*:
    a. Elevated potassium
    b. Elevated creatinine
    c. Elevated bicarbonate
    d. Elevated BUN
34. The specific gravity of Mr. Zanuck's urine has consistently been 1.010. This indicates:
    a. A normal, functioning kidney
    b. Loss of the kidneys' ability to concentrate urine
    c. That he is becoming dehydrated
    d. That he is anuric
35. Mr. Zanuck is placed on a low-protein, high-carbohydrate, low potassium, low sodium diet. Which of the following findings would reflect the desired therapeutic response of dietary restriction of protein?
    a. Blood pressure within normal limits
    b. Hemoglobin and hematocrit within normal limits
    c. Decreasing BUN and creatinine levels
    d. Phosphate levels within the normal range
36. Mr. Zanuck asks to have a snack because he was not hungry at lunch and did not eat. Which of the following would be appropriate?
    a. Bologna sandwich with milk
    b. Boiled egg, whole wheat toast, apple juice
    c. Grilled ham and cheese sandwich, blueberry muffin, tea
    d. Hot dog with bun, spinach salad, prunes, milk

Mr. Zanuck shows no signs of recovery. Peritoneal dialysis is initiated.

37. Nursing care of Mr. Zanuck while he is receiving peritoneal dialysis would include:
    a. Administering the dialysate at room temperature
    b. Infusing the dialysate over a 4-hour period
    c. Keeping a moist sterile dressing around the peritoneal catheter site
    d. Monitoring him for signs and symptoms of hypovolemia

38. The nurse infuses 2000 ml of dialysate and then clamps the tubing for 20 minutes. When the outflow tubing is unclamped to allow the fluid to drain from the peritoneal cavity, no drainage occurs. The nurse should:
  a. Connect the tubing to suction
  b. Notify the physician immediately
  c. Change the peritoneal catheter
  d. Turn the patient from side to side

39. The nurse would suspect that Mr. Zanuck is developing peritonitis when:
  a. Outflow from the third exchange is pink-tinged
  b. An elevated temperature and severe abdominal pain occur
  c. Abdominal distention occurs
  d. Hypotension and tachycardia occur

Mr. Zanuck never regains normal kidney function. He is discharged home on peritoneal dialysis. Four years later he is readmitted for a kidney transplant.

40. The most important requirement for the donated kidney to meet to minimize rejection reaction by Mr. Zanuck is:
  a. Histocompatibility
  b. ABO compatibility
  c. Mr. Zanuck's attitude toward the operation
  d. The age of the donor

41. Which of the following interventions will be used to prevent graft rejection in Mr. Zanuck following the kidney transplant?
  a. Administration of human leukocyte antigens
  b. Administration of Imuran and Cytoxan
  c. Placing him on reverse isolation
  d. Giving him an infusion of T-lymphocytes

42. The nurse would suspect that Mr. Zanuck is experiencing a rejection of the new kidney if:
  a. His blood pressure began to fall below normal range.
  b. He showed daily weight loss
  c. His urine output suddenly increased
  d. His serum creatinine showed a continual increase

43. Because he is receiving immunosuppressive therapy, Mr. Zanuck is prone to all of the following *except*:
  a. Leukopenia
  b. Alopecia
  c. Delayed wound healing
  d. Hypoglycemia

44. The kidney performs all of the following functions *except*:
  a. Regulation of blood pressure
  b. Control of body temperature
  c. Regulation of acid-base balance
  d. Erythropoiesis

45. What is the functional unit of the kidney?
  a. Glomeruli
  b. Collecting ducts
  c. Nephron
  d. Loop of Henle

46. When urine is finally excreted from the bladder, it is:
  a. Hypertonic
  b. Isotonic
  c. Hypotonic

47. The vast majority of electrolytes are reabsorbed in the:
    a. Bladder
    b. Collecting ducts
    c. Proximal convoluted tubules
    d. Bowman's capsule
48. Stimulation of the renin-angiotensin-aldosterone system causes:
    a. An increased production of red blood cells
    b. An increased urinary output
    c. An increased reabsorption of calcium and excretion of phosphates
    d. Increase in blood pressure
49. Which of the following questions should be used to assess whether a patient is experiencing hesitancy?
    a. "Do you have difficulty starting or maintaining your stream of urine?"
    b. "How frequently do you void?"
    c. "Do you experience the need to void immediately?"
    d. "Do you have difficulty controlling voiding?"
50. Since removal of his Foley catheter, Mr. Carter has been voiding small amounts (50-100 ml) frequently. The nurse should:
    a. Take no action for this is normal after removal of a Foley catheter
    b. Notify the physician immediately
    c. Encourage him to drink more fluids
    d. Ask him if he still feels the urge to void after voiding and then palpate his suprapubic area
51. Which of the following findings in a urinalysis would be abnormal?
    a. pH = 9.6
    b. Color = clear amber
    c. Protein = 0
    d. Sugar = 0

Mrs. Kelsey is alert, oriented, and ambulatory. She has an IV infusing into her right lower arm. Because she has been complaining of burning and pain with voiding, the physician orders a clean-catch urine for culture and sensitivity.

52. The nurse should:
    a. Catheterize Mrs. Kelsey to collect the urine specimen
    b. Give Mrs. Kelsey a sterile cup and have her void into it
    c. Instruct Mrs. Kelsey to cleanse with an antiseptic solution, void a small amount, stop, and then void into the sterile cup
    d. Cleanse Mrs. Kelsey herself and then have her void into the sterile specimen cup
53. The physician writes the following order: Catheterize for residual urine. If more than 75 ml leave catheter in place. The nurse should:
    a. Have the patient void, measure the output, insert a straight catheter, and measure the output
    b. Have the patient void, measure the output, insert a Foley catheter, and measure the output
    c. Insert a Foley catheter and connect it to a drainage bag
    d. Insert a straight catheter and measure the output

CASE STUDY I

Miss Kantor, a 26-year-old secretary, visits her doctor complaining of being tired most of the time, frequent headaches, and swelling of her feet. B/P = 210/124, P = 98, R = 24, T = 98.6° F. She is admitted to the hospital for diagnostic tests. The following results were obtained:

		Normal
Creatinine	= 18.5 mg/dl	0.5-1.5 mg/dl
Potassium	= 8.4 mEq/l	3.5-5.5 mEq/l
BUN	= 70 mg/dl	10-30 mg/dl
Sodium	= 94 mEq/l	135-145 mEq/l
Bicarbonate	= 12.0 mEq/l	20-30 mEq/l
Hemoglobin	= 8.4 g/dl	12.0-16.0 g/dl
Hematocrit	= 20%	35%-45%
Phosphorus	= 7.2 mg/dl	2.8-4.5 mg/dl

Urine specific gravity was 1.009 (normal is 1.010 to 1.030)

Miss Kantor indicates that she has had recurrent episodes of glomerulonephritis. A diagnosis of chronic renal failure is made.

A vascath is inserted in to her left subclavian vessel and she is started on hemodialysis twice a week. In addition to hemodialysis, the physician writes the following orders:

40 g protein, 2 g sodium, 40 mEq potassium diet
Amphogel 30 cc ml tid with meals
Catapres 0.1 mg bid
Daily weights
Activity as tolerated
Folic acid 1 tablet daily
Fluid restriction 1000 ml/day
Serum calcium level
No B/P or venipunctures in right arm

Two weeks later, Miss Kantor stabilizes with hemodialysis. An AV fistula is created in her right arm with use of a Gortex graft. She will be receiving hemodialysis on an outpatient basis at the local community dialysis center.

On her scheduled discharge day, the nurse finds Miss Kantor crying. When asked why she was crying, she responded, "Now I'll never be able to have sex again or have a baby."

1. Explain the pathophysiological basis for each of the clinical manifestations of chronic renal failure exhibited by Miss Kantor.

2. Explain the pathophysiological basis for each of the abnormal lab tests.

3. What is the rationale for each of the orders written by the physician?

4. What major problems could Miss Kantor experience during hemodialysis? What assessment parameters will be used to determine the effectiveness of hemodialysis?

5. What assessments should the nurse make to determine if the AV fistula is functioning normally?

6. What would be an appropriate response to Miss Kantor's statement about sexual functioning and pregnancy?

CASE STUDY II

Mrs. Mann was admitted to the hospital complaining of severe colicky pain in the left flank area. Urinalysis showed a moderate amount of RBCs, a large amount of WBCs, pus, and a bacteria count greater than 100,000/ml. An IVP revealed left hydronephrosis secondary to calculi lodged in the ureteropelvic junction. Laboratory analysis of the crystals found in the urine indicates calcium phosphate stones.

Mrs. Mann is scheduled to have shock-wave lithotripsy. An epidural block will be used for anesthesia. Ampicillin 1 Gm IV piggyback is ordered for her UTI. A primary IV of D_5W is ordered to be infused at 100 ml/hour. Additional orders include; Intake and output, strain all urine, Demerol 50-100 mg IM, q4h, prn for pain.

When the nurse enters the room to measure Mrs. Mann's urinary output total, Mrs. Mann states, "The doctor explained the type of procedure that was going to be used to get rid of my kidney stone so clearly, but it is a new procedure, and I'm feeling very nervous about it."

Two days after her UTI clears, she undergoes shock wave lithotripsy and returns to the clinical unit. The skin on the left midlateral area is red and tender.

Complete the care plan below. List two additional problems for the preoperative period and follow through on the care plan. For the postoperative period document one additional assessment and complete each column on the care plan.

Assessment	Nursing diagnosis	Goals	Interventions	Evaluation criteria
Preoperative Colicky pain in left flank area IVP shows hydronephrosis secondary to renal calculi	Pain: related to renal calculi			
Postoperative Had shock wave lithotripsy, epidural anesthesia				

CLINICAL ACTIVITIES

1. Examine the procedure manuals at your assigned clinical agency to determine the pre- and post-procedural care of the patient who undergoes the following diagnostic tests: cystoscopy, cystometrogram, IVP, retrograde pyelography, ultrasound, creatinine clearance, and renal biopsy.
2. Plan an observational experience in the departments where x-ray evaluations and direct visual tests of the urinary system are performed.
3. Where can patients with urinary diversions purchase stoma supplies in your community? How expensive are they?
4. What support groups are available in your community to help patients with urinary diversions adapt to altered body image?
5. Plan an observational experience with an enterostomal therapist (if one is available in your agency) or a home health care nurse who has to provide ostomy care to a patient at home with a urinary diversion stoma.
6. What support is available to the patient who is dying of endstage renal disease and their family? What is the most common cause of death in patients with chronic renal failure?
7. Visit a hemodialysis unit or center to observe what the nurse does with the patient before, during, and after dialysis.
8. Which form of dialysis is most popular in your community for long-term management of the chronic renal failure patient? Why?
9. What support is available in your community to help the patient and the family cope with chronic renal failure?
10. What is the incidence of chronic renal failure in your community? What are the most common causes of chronic renal failure in the patients in your community? How do your findings compare with national statistics?

SUGGESTED READINGS

Binkley, LS: Keeping up with peritoneal dialysis, Am J Nurs 84:729-733, June 1986.

The author describes persons who may be candidates for PD, how it works, how to prevent peritonitis, and how to recognize and deal with other associated complications such as pain, outflow problems, bloody effluent, tunnel infections, and nutrition.

Coleman, EA: When the kidney fails, RN 49:28-34, July 1986.

Engram, BW: Dos and don'ts of urologic nursing, Nursing 13:49, Oct 1983.

Pritchard, V: Geriatric infections; the urinary tract, RN 36-38, May 1988.

Solomon, J: Does renal failure mean sexual failure? RN 49:41-43, Aug 1986.

UNIT IX **Sexual and Reproductive Problems**

Chapter 33

Sexuality in Health and Illness

CAROLE KAUFMANN

CHAPTER OBJECTIVES

On completion of this chapter, the student should be able to:

- Describe changes that occur during the phases of human sexual response.
- Describe changes in sexuality that occur with aging.
- Differentiate types of sexual variation.
- Identify ways in which illness and environment affect sexuality.
- Identify types of alterations in sexual health and related nursing interventions.
- Describe methods of prevention of sexual problems.
- State approaches that facilitate assessment of sexual health.
- Describe levels of intervention for persons with alterations of sexual health.

PREREQUISITE READING

Long-Phipps, Chapter 33, pp. 1217-1237.

SELF-ASSESSMENT ACTIVITIES

I. Define the following terms.

Anal sexuality
Asexual
Cunnilingus
Excitement phase
Exhibitionism
Fellatio
Gender identity
Gender role
Grafenberg spot
Heterosexual
Homosexuality
Human sexuality
Kegel exercises
Phases of sexual response
Plateau phase
Resolution phase
Sexual frequency
Sexual function
Sexual health
Sexual relationships
Transvestism
Voyeurism
Zoophilia

II. Multiple choice

1. Masters and Johnson pioneered the scientific study of which of the following aspects of sexual behavior?
   - **a.** Holistic
   - **b.** Physiologic
   - **c.** Ethical
   - **d.** Gender identity
2. Sexual tension becomes intensified during which of the following phases of sexual response?
   - **a.** Orgasm
   - **b.** Excitement
   - **c.** Plateau
   - **d.** Resolution
3. Vaginal lubrication appears early in sexual stimulation.
   - **a.** True
   - **b.** False

4. The vaginal barrel becomes enlarged and wider during which phase of the sexual reponse?
   a. Excitement
   b. Orgasm
   c. Plateau
   d. Resolution
5. During the excitement phase, the nipples of male and female breasts become erect.
   a. True
   b. False
6. The plateau phase is characterized by:
   a. Sexual tension
   b. Intense vasocongestion of genitalia
   c. Release of sexual tension
   d. Uterine contractions
7. Orgasm involves which of the following?
   a. Propulsion of semen backwards into the male bladder
   b. Intense uterine contractions
   c. Increase in vasoconstriction
   d. Vasomotor ataxia
8. An important fact for U.S. health professionals to remember is that:
   a. There are many variations of sexual behavior
   b. Most variations in sexual behavior are tolerated in this society
   c. Homosexuals are typically sexually hyperactive
   d. Precopulatory stimulation should be avoided
9. Bisexuality may be defined as:
   a. Choice of adult sexual partner of opposite sex
   b. Choice of adult sexual partner of same sex
   c. Choice of adult sexual partner of same and opposite sex
   d. Sexual relations with close relative
10. The physiologic mechanism of sexual dysfunction in a young man with a spinal cord injury of C5:
    a. Disrupts integrity of peripheral nerves and spinal cord reflexes involved in sexual response
    b. Interferes with function of centers controlling sexual drive
    c. Interferes with hormonal balance
    d. Interferes with comfort during intercourse
11. During your nursing assessment, you ascertain that Mrs. Jones, a diabetic, is experiencing dyspareunia. What additional assessment should be made before a nursing diagnosis and interventions are made?
    a. Assess for frequency of intercourse
    b. Assess for phimosis
    c. Assess for gaping vaginal opening
    d. Assess for adequate vaginal lubrication

Mrs. Procter, 34, had a hysterectomy 2 days ago. She and her husband have three children. Her concerns beyond her postoperative period are for her relationship with her husband, how the operation will affect her femininity, how to cope with surgical menopause, and its effect on her body functions. The nurse validates Mrs. Procter's concerns and says, "Shall we talk about your concerns?"

12. Mrs. Procter asks the nurse about her physical relationship with her husband. The nurse realizes that Mrs. Procter's concerns are focused on:
    a. Her recent surgery
    b. Her ability to feel sexual desire
    c. Her self-image and self-concept
    d. Her husband's feelings about her body changes
13. Probable nursing diagnoses for Mrs. Procter would be:
    a. Body image disturbance
    b. Sexual dysfunction
    c. Altered sexual patterns
    d. All of above

14. Mrs. Procter expresses concern also about her ability to have satisfying sexual intercourse and asks her nurse about this. The best reply the nurse could make is:
    a. "Your concern is about your ability to enjoy your sexual relationship because of your physical capabilities?"
    b. "You don't seem to think your husband will enjoy sex?"
    c. "What exactly is your primary concern?"
    d. "Thus far, how exactly is your relationship with your husband?"
15. The *first* appropriate nursing intervention for Mrs. Procter is:
    a. A sexual health assessment
    b. Referral to her physician
    c. Referral to a sexual counselor
    d. All of the above
16. For an interview relating to sexual health assessment, the nurse should *first:*
    a. Ask Mrs. Procter when she wants to discuss her concerns
    b. Create an appropriate setting for the interview
    c. Make an appointment for her husband to be present
    d. Make an appointment for her surgeon to be present
17. Which of the following is not a type of sexual dysfunction?
    a. Alterations in sexual desire
    b. Alterations in orgasm
    c. Alterations of arousal
    d. Alterations in sexual partners
18. A low sexual desire can result from all of the following factors *except:*
    a. Low androgen levels
    b. Lack of sexual teaching
    c. Depression
    d. Drugs
19. Penile implants are used in the treatment of which type of sexual dysfunction arising from a pathophysiologic basis?
    a. Alterations in vasocongestion
    b. Alterations in orgasm
    c. Alterations in arousal
    d. All of the above
20. Alterations in orgasm include problems with:
    a. Ejaculatory function
    b. Erection
    c. Dyspareunia
    d. Low sexual desire
21. One of the primary causes of premature ejaculation is:
    a. Premature penile development
    b. Overuse of certain drugs
    c. Physical immaturity
    d. Anxiety
22. A patient has had a left radical mastectomy. The most significant nursing problem for this patient would be:
    a. Alterations in orgasm
    b. Alterations in arousal
    c. Alterations in body image
    d. Alterations in sexual functioning
23. Mr. Simpson has approached you as a nurse and begins to tell you that he feels that he is trapped in the body of a man. This patient wishes to discuss his feelings. The definition of his problem is:
    a. Hermaphoditism
    b. Transvestism
    c. Anorgasm
    d. Transsexualism

24. The prerequisites for nursing practice in the area of sexual counseling include all of the following *except:*
    a. Awareness of surgical procedures
    b. Awareness of own value system
    c. Ability to communicate
    d. A knowledge base
25. Education of patient population implies more than mere dissemination of information. To be more effective, the nurse should encourage the patient to:
    a. Tell the nurse what he or she learned in school
    b. Explore his or her attitudes regarding sex
    c. Read several pamphlets on sex
    d. Undergo surgery

SUGGESTED READINGS

Foltz, AT: The influence of cancer on self-concept and life quality (review), Semin Oncol Nurs 3,4:303-312, Nov 1987.

McKenzie, F: Sexuality after total pelvic exenteration Nurs Times 84(20):26-28, May 18-24, 1988.

Steinke, EE: Older adults knowledge and attitudes about sexuality and aging (research), Image Nurs Sch 20(2):93-95, Summer 1988.

Wood, SL: Facing the reality of teen sex, Physician Assist 12(6):138, Jun 1988.

Chapter 34

The Patient with Reproductive Problems

CAROLE KAUFMANN

CHAPTER OBJECTIVES

On completion of this chapter, the student should be able to:

- Describe measures for prevention of genital infections and early detection of cancer.
- Identify health teaching regarding menstruation and menopause.
- Describe methods and effects of sterilization, and assessment methods and counseling for infertility.
- Describe the types and effects of inflammatory and structural disorders of the reproductive tract in females and males.
- Identify the incidence and different sites of cancer of the reproductive tract in females and males.
- Describe nursing care for persons experiencing surgery of the reproductive tract.

PREREQUISITE READING

Long-Phipps, Chapter 34, pp. 1239-1278.

SELF-ASSESSMENT ACTIVITIES

I. Using the following words, label the anatomic diagram of the female reproductive tract on the following page.

Urethral orifice
Labium majora
Clitoris
Cervix
Uterus
Ovary
Vagina
Fallopian tube
Labium minora
Frenulum of labia

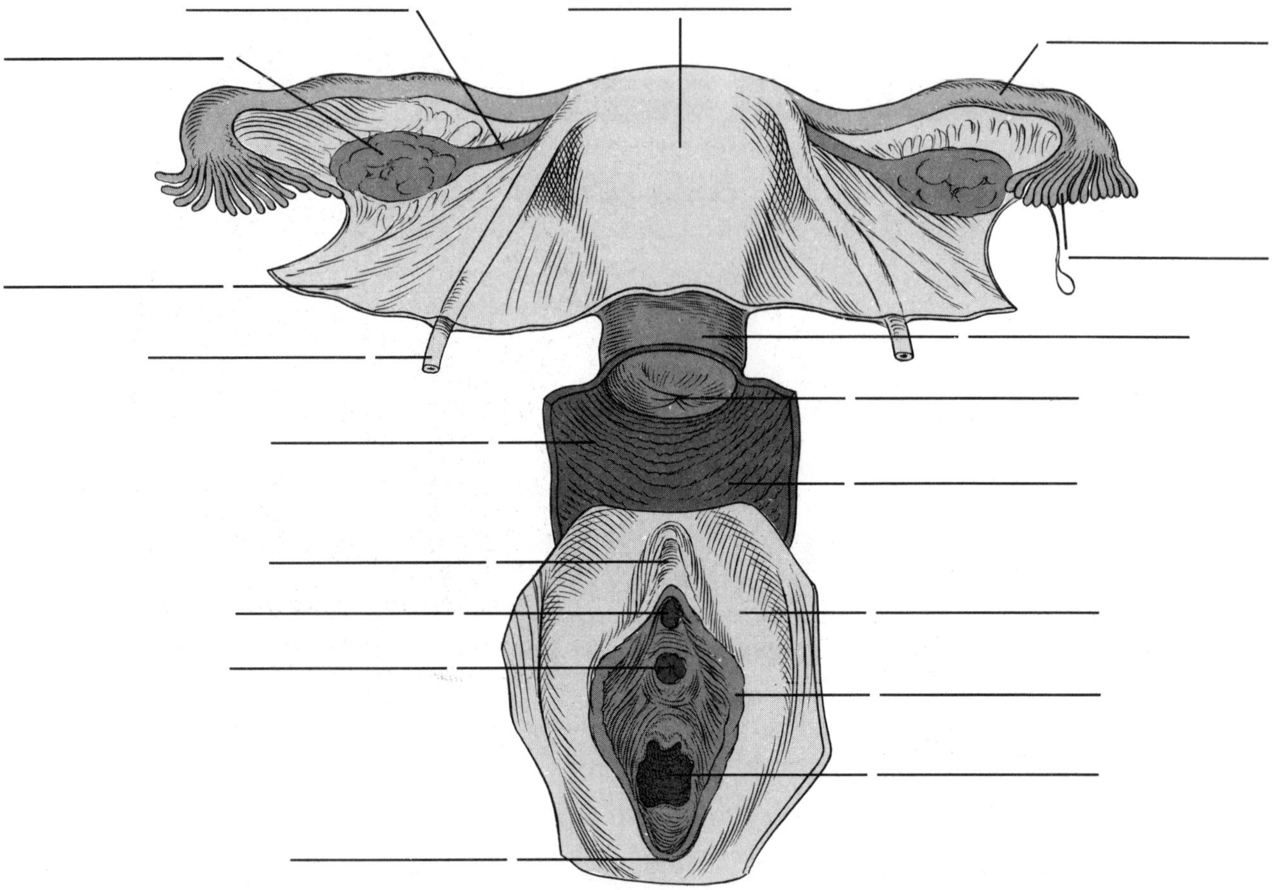

II. Using the following words, label the anatomic diagram of the male reproductive tract on the following page.

Epididymis
Glans penis
Prepuce (foreskin)
Prostate gland
Bladder
Seminal vesicle and duct
Scrotum
Testis
Vas deferens

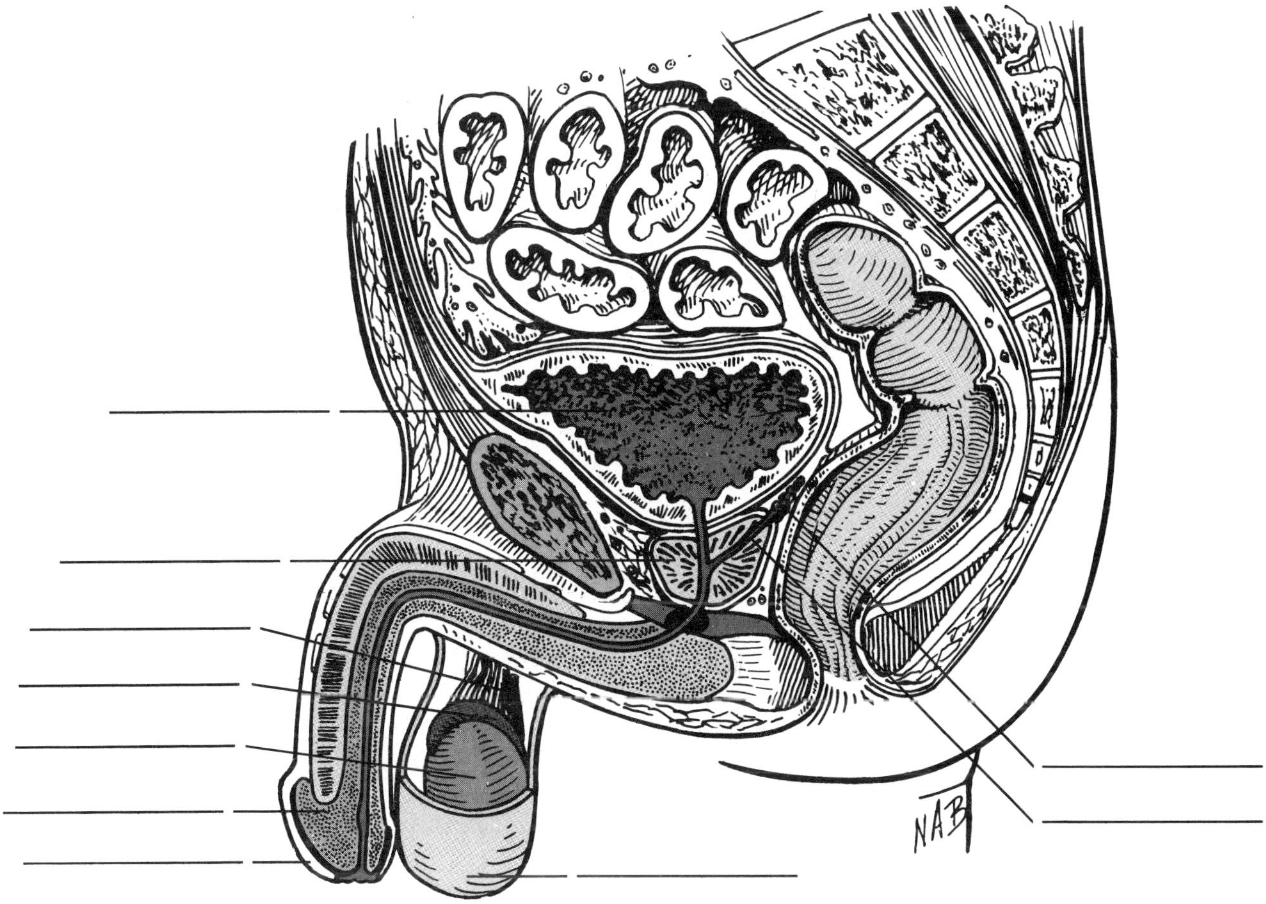

III. Multiple choice

1. During the period before puberty and after menopause, females are at greater risk for developing vaginal infections because:
   a. The vaginal epithelium is thicker
   b. The vaginal pH is more acid
   c. The vaginal pH is alkaline
   d. The introitus of the vagina is narrower
2. The major hormones produced by the ovaries are:
   a. Estrogen and luteinizing hormones
   b. Progesterone and lactogenic hormone
   c. Follicule-stimulating hormone and luteinizing hormone
   d. Estrogen and progesterone
3. During the secretory phase of the menstrual cycle the following takes place:
   a. Formation of the corpus luteum
   b. Development of the mature graffian follicle
   c. Shedding of endometrial lining
   d. Secretion of follicle-stimulating hormone
4. Methods of preventing vaginal infections include all of the following *except:*
   a. Voiding shortly after intercourse
   b. Wiping from front to back after bowel movements
   c. Frequent douching
   d. Using a condom during intercourse

5. In health teaching about menstruation for a young teenager, the nurse should include:
   a. Avoiding tub baths
   b. Decreasing activity to prevent discomfort
   c. Wearing a pad during early period of heavy flow
   d. Increasing salt intake to conserve fluids
6. The first day of the menstrual cycle begins:
   a. On the first day of menstrual flow
   b. On the last day of menstrual flow
   c. When the ovum is released into the fallopian tubes
   d. When the pituitary gland secretes follicle-stimulating hormone (FSH)
7. Which of the following statements about a Pap smear is *not* correct?
   a. The test cannot be performed during menstruation.
   b. Patients should douche before the test.
   c. Two specimens are taken from the cervix.
   d. The specimens are smeared on a glass slide and a fixative is applied.
8. Premenstrual syndrome (PMS) occurs in more than 25% of menstruating women. The symptoms occur as a result of:
   a. Changes in hormones only
   b. Psychologic changes
   c. Changes in glucose tolerance
   d. Changes in hormone levels and altered glucose tolerance
9. Some of the measures to relieve dysmenorrhea are:
   a. Manual pressure on abdomen
   b. Muscle toning
   c. Breathing techniques
   d. All of the above
10. The most common method of voluntary birth control for couples over age 30 is:
   a. Diaphragm
   b. Tubal ligation
   c. Vasectomy
   d. Birth control pill
11. Which of the following endoscopic procedures involves use of a local anesthetic, after which a small incision is created in near the umbilicus through which a metal instrument is inserted and the cavity insufflated with carbon dioxide for visualization of all pelvic organs?
   a. Colposcopy
   b. Culdoscopy
   c. Laparoscopy
   d. Hysteroscopy
12. The procedure for doing a vasectomy includes:
   a. Tying of vas deferens through a scrotal incision
   b. Removal of epididymis through a scrotal incision
   c. Removal of a segment of vas deferens through a scrotal incision
   d. Removal of a segment of prostate through scrotal incision
13. Teaching for the patient who has had a vasectomy include:
   a. Continue to use another birth control method
   b. Wear tight jockey-type shorts
   c. Apply warm compresses to scrotum immediately
   d. Resume sexual activity as soon as it is comfortable without need of additional birth control
14. In treating an infertile couple with a diagnosis of oligospermia, the treatment of choice would be:
   a. Injection of Clomid to the mother
   b. Fallopian tube insufflation
   c. Surrogate mother
   d. Heterologous artificial insemination

15. In assessing the patient with a vaginal infection described as yellow to green, frothy, foul-smelling, and copious, the medical diagnosis would be:
    a. Trichomonas
    b. Trichinosis
    c. Candida
    d. Gardnerella
16. The nursing diagnosis would include knowledge deficit. The implementation would include assisting with achievement of therapeutic goals. The medication of choice would be:
    a. Monostat vaginal cream
    b. Nystatin vaginal cream
    c. Sodium bicarbonate vaginal douche
    d. Metronidazole (Flagyl) orally
17. Toxic shock during menstruation may be prevented by:
    a. Frequent changing of vulvar pad
    b. Avoidance of superabsorbent tampons
    c. Douching following menstruation
    d. Leaving tampon in place at least 8 hours to avoid lesions in the vagina

In assessing Mrs. Smith, a 34-year-old obese woman, the nurse practitioner ascertains that she has a vaginal discharge. On pelvic examination, the nurse notes a white, curdlike, cheesy discharge with a sweetish odor.

18. The most likely diagnosis is:
    a. Candida
    b. Trichomonas
    c. Chlamydia
    d. Gardnerella
19. In doing a complete assessment, the nurse practitioner would include:
    a. An HGB and Hct to rule out anemia
    b. A T3, T4 to rule out thyroid disease
    c. A GTT to rule out diabetes mellitus
    d. An ELISA to rule out AIDS
20. The drug that would be prescribed for this condition is:
    a. Ampicillin orally
    b. Monistat vaginally
    c. Flagyl orally
    d. Tetracycline orally
21. Mrs. Frank is a 55-year-old woman who complains to you of urinary incontinence, especially when she coughs or laughs. She is scheduled for surgery next week, and you are instructed to teach Mrs. Frank Kegel exercises. The most effective method of teaching Mrs. Frank how to do Kegel exercises is:
    a. Place a finger along the upper vaginal wall while tightening the perineum
    b. Place the palm of your hand over the abdomen while tightening the abdominal muscles
    c. Place your hands over the gluteal muscles while tightening the gluteal maximus muscle
    d. Knee-chest position for 5 minutes three times a day

Mrs. Peters is a 35-year-old woman with a history of endometriosis. She is complaining of severe pain during menstruation, dyspareunia, and irregular periods.

22. The pathophysiology of this condition is:
    a. The ovaries are polycystic and may become malignant
    b. The tubes have become occluded as a result of PID
    c. Endometrial cells are seeded in surrounding tissues and bleed during menstruation
    d. The uterus is prolapsed as a result of childbirth injury
23. Conservative treatment of endometriosis may include:
    a. A pessary to support the uterus
    b. Oral contraceptives to decrease the amount of menstrual flow
    c. Ampicillin
    d. Metronidazole vaginal suppositories

24. The conservative treatment does not work, so Mrs. Peters is scheduled to have a hysterectomy. The nurse should prepare Mrs. Peters (expecting radical hysterectomy) by explaining:
    a. The possible complications and prognosis
    b. Postoperative care she can expect
    c. Postoperative abdominal distention
    d. Feelings of postoperative grief or loss
25. Which of the following is not recommended for a postoperative hysterectomy patient?
    a. Antiembolic stockings to knee
    b. Allowed out of bed the day of surgery
    c. Lowering head of bed to flat position for a short time every 2 hours for 24 hours
    d. A pillow under the knees
26. Which of the discharge instructions below is not appropriate for a postoperative hysterectomy patient?
    a. You can wear a girdle
    b. Avoid heavy lifting for 2 months
    c. Avoid dancing for 1 month after discharge
    d. Resume sexual intercourse in 4 to 6 weeks
27. Mrs. Rogers is quiet and depressed 4 days after her hysterectomy and tells the nurse she is worried about her husband's responses to her surgery. The nurse should respond:
    a. "You have already had two children, why are you worried?"
    b. "You should follow your surgeon's instructions, but usually sexual intercourse can be resumed in 3 to 4 months."
    c. "Don't feel guilty, it's not your fault."
    d. "We can discuss your usual activities associated with your femininity."
28. Mrs. Burkes, a 48-year-old saleswoman, has just been notified by her gynecologist that her cervical Pap smear indicated stage II carcinoma. This means:
    a. Confined to cervix
    b. Extends outside cervix, but does not involve pelvic wall
    c. Involves pelvic wall and lower third of vagina
    d. Involves bladder and rectum
29. Mrs. Burkes and her doctor participate in a treatment plan that includes radiotherapy. Some of the problems that may occur following pelvic irradiation are:
    a. Loss of hair
    b. Feeling of greatly expanded vagina
    c. Lack of libido
    d. Hydrocele

IV. Complete the following chart on benign tumors of the female genital tract.

Epidemiology	Pathophysiology and diagnostic tests	Clinical picture	Describe perioperative care of woman undergoing hysterectomy
Ovarian tumors and cysts			
Fibroid tumors			
Endometriosis			
Cervical polyps			

V. Summarize the major facts regarding cancer of the female genital tract in the space provided.

Cancer of the cervix

Epidemiology and etiology

Prevention and early detection

Clinical picture, diagnostic tests

Intervention

Stages of cervical cancer

Stage	Involvement	Treatment option
0		
I		
II		
III		
IV		

VI. Complete the following chart.

STD	Etiology and epidemiology	Pathophysiology and diagnostic tests	Clinical manifestations	Treatment
Chlamydial infection				
Men				
Women				
Lympogranuloma venereum				
Gardnerella vaginitis				
Chancroid				

Continued

STD	Etiology and epidemiology	Pathophysiology and diagnostic tests	Clinical manifestations	Treatment
Donovanosis				
Trichomoniasis				
Candidiasis				

VII. Complete the chart below.

	Etiology and epidemiology	Pathophysiology and diagnostic tests	Clinical manifestations	Treatment
Prostatitis				
Epididymitis				

VII. Fill in the chart below on prostatic neoplasm and neoplasms of the testes and penis.

	Testes	Prostate	Penis
Etiology			
Diagnosis			
Clinical picture and diagnostic tests			
Staging			

Continued

	Testes	Prostate	Penis
Interventions			
Postoperative care			
Complications			

IX. Summarize the pertinent data concerning the following conditions of the male reproductive system. Include diagnostic tests.

1. Phimosis
2. Paraphimosis
3. Orchitis
4. Hydrocele
5. Stermatocele
6. Varicocele
7. Priapism
8. Torsion of the testes

SUGGESTED READINGS

Bosi, GJ: Detecting testicular cancer early, Emerg Med 20(9):34-37, 39-40, 1988.
McDonie, TM: Pain location: reports by abdominal hysterectomy patients, (research), Fla Nurse 36(5):5, 1988.
Pediatric management problems (case study), Pediatr Nurs 14(4):346-347, 1988.

Chapter 35

Sexually Transmitted Diseases

CAROLE KAUFMANN

CHAPTER OBJECTIVES

On completion of this chapter, the student should be able to:

- Define sexually transmitted diseases (STDs).
- Describe the transmission, prevention, and control of STDs.
- List the causative agent, incubation period, signs and symptoms, medical therapy, and long-term effects of gonorrhea, syphilis, herpes genitalis, and chlamydia infection.
- Describe the subjective and objective data to be collected from a person suspected of having an STD.
- Write a teaching plan for a unit on the prevention of STDs for a sex education course for adolescents.

PREREQUISITE READING

Long-Phipps, Chapter 35, pp. 1279-1301.

SELF-ASSESSMENT ACTIVITIES

I. Multiple choice

1. Sexually transmitted diseases can be transmitted from one person to another by:
- **a.** The toilet seat
- **b.** Shaking hands
- **c.** Contact with genitalia, mouth, or rectum
- **d.** The doorknob

2. The people who are at risk for STDs are:
- **a.** Only prostitutes
- **b.** Only homosexuals
- **c.** Only single men
- **d.** All sexually active individuals

3. One of the better ways of preventing transmissions of an STD is:
- **a.** Use of mechanical barrier such as condom
- **b.** Vaginal douching
- **c.** Do not open any doors with doorknobs
- **d.** Do not borrow anyone else's clothes

4. In planning prevention and control measures for STD, there are three levels of prevention. The first level is:
- **a.** Preventing the disease
- **b.** Prevention of complications
- **c.** Decreasing effects of complications
- **d.** Contact investigation

5. When teaching the proper use of condoms, you should include all of the following points *except:*
- **a.** Condoms should be stored in a cool, dry place
- **b.** Put condom on tightly from the tip to the base
- **c.** Use only water-based lubricants
- **d.** Hold condom in place while withdrawing still-erect penis from vagina

John Buchanan, a 42-year-old lawyer, comes into STD clinic with a complaint of a purulent discharge from his urethra.

6. In doing an assessment, the nurse would question John about all of the following *except*:
   a. Sexual orientation
   b. Number of sexual partners
   c. Rectal symptoms
   d. Dietary patterns

7. One of the doctors suspects that John has gonorrhea. One of the diagnostic tests that would be used is:
   a. Blood serologic test
   b. Biopsy of penis
   c. Smear of discharge for culture
   d. Fern test

8. The treatment of choice of gonorrhea, assuming that John has no allergies, is:
   a. Ampicillin
   b. Tetracycline
   c. Cryotherapy
   d. Erythromysin

Maryann Dorsay is a 24-year-old pregnant woman whose ED is 10 days. She complains today of pain and inflammation in the perineal area. She also mentions that she has headaches and flulike symptoms. On inspection of the perineum you note multiple reddish papules and clear, fluid-filled vesicles on her vagina and perineum. The doctor diagnoses genital herpes, confirmed by isolation of herpes genitalis from the lesions.

9. The doctor discusses the mode of delivery. The baby's estimated weight is 6 lb. The most likely method will be:
   a. Cesarean section
   b. Spontaneous labor with vaginal delivery
   c. Induction with vaginal delivery

10. To prevent spread of herpes to the family members, Maryann is taught to:
   a. Eat alone with separate utensils
   b. Use separate towels
   c. Douche before having intercourse
   d. Come to the clinic for penicillin

II. Complete the following chart on sexually transmitted diseases.

Disease process	Epidemiology, etiology, and prevention	Pathophysiology and diagnostic tests	Clinical manifestations	Interventions
Gonorrhea				
Syphilis				
Herpes genitalis				
Chlamydia				
Condylomata accuminata				

Continued

Disease process	Epidemiology, etiology, and prevention	Pathophysiology and diagnostic tests	Clinical manifestations	Interventions
Hepatitis A				
Lice				
Candidiasis				
Gardnerella vaginilis				
Trichomoniasis				
AIDS (see text)				

III. Complete the following nursing assessment of Mr. Jones, a patient with the STD gonorrhea.

Assessment	Nursing diagnosis	Intervention	Evaluation
Subjective data			
Objective data			
Diagnostic tests			

CLINICAL ACTIVITY

Plan a complete teaching guide on STDs for a class of high school freshmen. Include all teaching aids and handouts to be used. Suggestion: Go to your local health department for teaching aids and information.

SUGGESTED READINGS

Dalgeish, AG, and others: Surgical gloves as a mechanical barrier against human immuno deficiency viruses (research), Br J Surg 75(2):171-172, 1988.

Northrap, CE: Rights versus regulation: confidentiality in the age of AIDS, Nurs Outlook 36(4):208, 1988.

Schofferman, J: Hospice care of the patient with AIDS, Hospice J 3(4):51-74, 1987.

Stover, S: New study to offer Zividine to HIV exposed health workers, Am Med News, 11, June 10, 1988.

Turner, JG, and others: Preventing HIV transmission in health care settings, AAOHN J 36(7):254-257, 1988.

Wilson, D: An overview of sexually transmitted diseases in the perinatal period, J Nurse Midwifery 33(3):115-128, 1988.

Chapter 36

The Patient with Problems of the Breast

CAROLE KAUFMANN

CHAPTER OBJECTIVES

On completion of this chapter, the student should be able to:

- Describe breast self-examination (guidelines, techniques).
- Explain diagnostic tests for breast evaluation.
- Differentiate between benign and malignant breast disorders.
- Describe the pathophysiology and interventions for women with benign breast disorders.
- Describe the risk factors and pathophysiology of breast cancer.
- Describe the types of surgery for breast cancer, most common procedures, and postoperative care.
- Describe types of breast reconstruction and required care.

PREREQUISITE READING

Long-Phipps, Chapter 36, pp.1303-1324.

SELF-ASSESSMENT ACTIVITIES

I. Define the following terms.

ERA
Fibroadenomas
Gynecomastia
Mastitis
Oophorectomy
Orange peel effect

II. Multiple choice

1. Women who complain of premenstrual breast discomfort should be counseled to:
   a. Decrease physical activity and get extra rest
   b. Increase physical activity
   c. Increase potassium intake
   d. Take off bra to lessen constriction of breast
2. Mammography is about 90% accurate in diagnosing early breast cancer in:
   a. Adolescents
   b. Nulliparous women
   c. Multiparous women
   d. Large-breasted women
3. The best time to perform the breast self-examination (BSE) each month is:
   a. First day of menstruation
   b. In the middle of the cycle
   c. 3 to 4 days after the conclusion of the menstrual flow
   d. 7 to 8 days after the conclusion of the menstrual flow

4. All women should begin breast self-examination:
   a. At high school age
   b. At 20 years of age
   c. After first baby
   d. After 40 years of age
5. When teaching breast self-examination, the individual should be instructed to do all of the following *except:*
   a. Use a systematic approach
   b. Examine the entire breast, including the tail and nipple
   c. Use the palm of the hand for palpation
   d. Perform the examination in a supine and erect position
6. There are several dietary aids that may be helpful in reducing symptoms of mammary dysplasia. They are:
   a. Avoid lean beef, pork, and chicken
   b. Avoid coffee, tea, and chocolate
   c. Avoid table salt, pretzels, and potato chips
   d. Avoid vitamins A and D

Betty Coffenne, a young single female, is admitted to the hospital for a right modified radical mastectomy. Surgery is scheduled for the next morning.

7. Which of the following questions would be of least importance to ask at this time?
   a. "How do you feel about having a mastectomy?"
   b. "Do you have a male friend with whom you are intimately involved?"
   c. "How long have you been performing breast self-examination?"
   d. "What effect do you think the mastectomy will have on your life?"
8. When Betty initially returns to the clinical unit following a mastectomy, exercises are started to prevent muscle stiffness and contracture of the shoulder. Initially, she should be instructed to:
   a. Move both arms as if pulling a rope
   b. Bend forward from the waist and swing both arms in a circular motion
   c. Brush teeth and hair with the arm on the operative side
   d. Flex and extend the fingers, then supinate and pronate the forearm
9. Two major long-term adaptive problems that result from a mastectomy are:
   a. Altered body image and loss
   b. Lymphedema and pain
   c. Infection and social isolation
   d. Immobility and alterations in nutrition
10. Following a mastectomy, the patient may be fitted for a breast prosthesis:
    a. On the day of discharge from the hospital
    b. When the incision is healed
    c. When she is able to perform full ROM with the arm on the operative side
    d. Whenever she expresses a need for one
11. All of the following manifestations are indicative of advanced breast cancer *except:*
    a. Occasional clear fluid discharge from the nipple
    b. Puckering of the skin
    c. Changes in skin color
    d. Progressive inversion of the nipple
12. The final decision as to what type of treatment program the patient will follow is made by:
    a. The physician
    b. The patient
    c. The nurse
    d. The insurance company

13. To prevent lymphedema of the arm on the side of the mastectomy, the nurse should do all of the following *except:*
    a. Elevate the arm
    b. Use the arm on the unaffected side for blood pressures
    c. Apply an ice pack and elastic bandage
    d. Avoid using the arm for blood drawings and injections
14. Following a modified radical mastectomy, a patient returns to the clinical unit with a Hemovac in place. The primary purpose of the Hemovac is to:
    a. Prevent the need for early dressing changes
    b. Prevent lymphedema
    c. Prevent the need for sutures
    d. Prevent hematoma formation
15. Which statement about interstitial radiation therapy is incorrect?
    a. The patient is usually treated on an outpatient basis.
    b. Radioactive needles are implanted into the breast tissue under local anesthesia.
    c. The patient requires isolation.
    d. The needles remain in place for about 3 days and then they are removed by the physician.
16. Which of the following statements about mammoplasty is correct?
    a. All mastectomy patients should be encouraged to have a mammoplasty.
    b. The goal of mammoplasty is to make the mastectomee whole again.
    c. Mammoplasty does not prevent postmastectomy depression.
    d. Mammoplasty can only be performed after the mastectomy wound has healed.
17. The primary reason that some patients who have malignant breast cancer may also require an oophorectomy or adrenalectomy later is:
    a. To remove the sources of estrogen and thereby retard the spread of the tumor
    b. To prevent or minimize the patient's stress reaction to the diagnosis of breast cancer
    c. To prevent the patient from having a menstrual period, which can be an additional source of anxiety
    d. Because these are the primary sites to which metastasis usually occurs
18. The treatment program for breast cancer is primarily dependent upon:
    a. What the patient wants and feels is the best
    b. Any of the latest therapies documented in magazines
    c. The patient's socioeconomic level
    d. The stage and TNM classification of the tumor
19. The test used to determine whether a breast tumor is benign or malignant is:
    a. Mammogram
    b. Thermography
    c. Ultrasonography
    d. Biopsy
20. The primary mode of metastasis of malignant breast cells is:
    a. Blood vessels
    b. Direct contact
    c. Unknown
    d. Lymphatic vessels
21. When a breast biopsy is performed, a hormone assay test is also performed on a sample of the tissue to:
    a. Determine whether the cancer cells are estrogen dependent
    b. Determine what the patient's estrogen levels is
    c. Determine the amount of progesterone replacement therapy needed
    d. Determine what the patient's progesterone level is
22. Mortality from breast cancer can be prevented by:
    a. Breast self-examination
    b. Using combination chemotherapy to treat breast cancer
    c. Performing radical mastectomies instead of modified radical mastectomies
    d. Using radiation after all mastectomies

23. The primary reason that breast self-examination is recommended to be performed monthly is:
    - **a.** So that the person will not forget the steps involved in the examination
    - **b.** So that the person will have a better awareness of what healthy breast tissue feels like
    - **c.** That it takes about 1 year for the person to feel comfortable in performing the examination
    - **d.** That breast tumors are insidious and metastasize very rapidly
24. Postmenopausal women should be instructed to perform breast self-examination:
    - **a.** On the same date of their choice each month
    - **b.** On a different date of their choice each month
    - **c.** Every day, because they are at high risk for breast cancer
    - **d.** Whenever they begin to take estrogen supplements
25. A simple mastectomy includes:
    - **a.** Removal of tumor mass and 2.5 to 7.5 cm of surrounding tissue
    - **b.** Removal of all underlying breast tissue, leaving skin, areola and nipple intact
    - **c.** Removal of entire breast but not axillary nodes
    - **d.** Complete removal of breast and removal of some axillary lymph nodes
26. The primary cause of nonmalignant breast diseases in the male and female is:
    - **a.** Trauma to the breast
    - **b.** Excessive manipulation of the breast
    - **c.** Estrogen imbalance
    - **d.** Delayed puberty

III. Complete the chart on malignant breast disorders.

	Dysplasia	**Fibroadenomas**	**Gynecomastia**
Prominent findings			
Distribution (unilateral or bilateral)			
Incidence			
Treatment			
Risk for becoming malignant			

CASE STUDY

Chrissy Bennett, age 34, never performed routine breast self-examination, although she had been taught the procedure 18 years ago after her first child was born. She has two teenage daughters.

On a visit to her doctor's office for an employment physical, the doctor discovered a large, hard, nonpliable lump in the lateral aspect of her left breast. A mammogram revealed findings indicative of cancer. She was admitted to the hospital for a biopsy that confirmed metastatic breast cancer, stage II. A total body scan was done to determine the extent of metastasis.

A left modified radical mastectomy was performed 2 days after the biopsy. Following surgery, she returns to the clinical unit with a Hemovac in place. The physician orders progressive resistance exercises to her left arm and the left arm kept elevated.

Although her husband makes a daily visit to see her at the hospital, she suspects that his feelings toward her have changed. At home he would embrace her with a passionate kiss, but since her mastectomy he seems reluctant to touch her. He only kisses her lightly on the forehead.

One day when her daughters visit, they ask the nurse, "Does this mean that we'll get breast cancer since our mom has it?"

1. In the premenopausal female, why is breast self-examination not recommended to be performed at the beginning of the menstrual period?

2. What are the three primary sites of metastasis with breast cancer?

3. What would be an appropriate response to the question posed by Mrs. Bennett's daughters?

4. When should arm exercises be started? What type of arm exercises should she be taught on a progressive exercise program? What is the purpose of exercises?

5. Is there a need for Mrs. Bennett to be taught breast self-examination? If so, what instructions would you give her?

6. What is the earliest sign of cancer of the breast?

7. What risk factors related to breast cancer should the nurse ask Mrs. Bennett about when taking a nursing history during the preoperative period?

8. What are some common factors that may influence Mrs. Bennett's psychological reaction to a mastectomy?

DIRECTIONS FOR RESEARCH

How can preoperative preparation of the mastectomy patient be improved? Design a simple questionnaire and administer it to mastectomy patients. For example, the questionnaire may ask:

1. "Do you feel you were adequately prepared to cope with a mastectomy before surgery?"

2. "If you answered no to the above question, what do you feel should have been done before surgery to better prepare you to deal with the problems you have experienced since your mastectomy?"

CLINICAL ACTIVITIES

1. What is the incidence of breast cancer among premenopausal and postmenopausal women in your community? Consult surgeons who perform mastectomies in your community or check the medical records department of local hospitals for these data.
2. What treatment protocols are being used in your community for the different stages of breast cancer? What is the prevalence of each stage in your community?
3. What agencies or organizations are available in your community to provide psychosocial support to the mastectomy patient? What services are provided by each? What is the process involved in referring patients to these services?
4. Where can patients purchase special mastectomy bras? How expensive are they?
5. Use the technique of breast self-examination, as outlined by the American Cancer Society (pp. 1304-1305 in Long-Phipps), to examine your own breast.
6. Teach breast self-examination to your next female patient.

SUGGESTED READINGS

Bunn, JC, and others: Reduction mammoplasty: the laser deepitheliazation technique (pictorial), AORN J 48(1):50-51, 1988.

Haughey, BP, and others: Breast self-examination: reported practices, proficiency, and stage of disease at diagnosis (research), Oncol Nurs Form 15(3): 315-319, 1988.

Williams, RD, and others: Barriers to breast cancer screening in older women, Fam Commun Health 10(3):51-56, 1987.

Chapter 37

Biologic Defense Mechanisms of the Human Body

BRENDA GOODNER

CHAPTER OBJECTIVES

On completion of this chapter, the student should be able to:

- Differentiate between the concepts of self and nonself.
- Identify the external and internal nonspecific biologic defense mechanisms.
- Define the steps of the inflammatory process, containment of infection, and resolution of inflammation.
- Explain the bases for the five cardinal signs of inflammation.
- Define antigens and antibodies and describe the antigen-antibody interactions.
- Differentiate between B cells and T cells and describe the humoral and cell-mediated responses to antigens.
- Explain the immunologic bases for passive and active immunizations, cancer, AIDS, and tissue transplantation.

PREREQUISITE READING

Long-Phipps, Chapter 37, pp. 1327-1352

SELF-ASSESSMENT ACTIVITIES

I. Define the following terms.

Absolute immunity
Acquired immunity
Active immunity
Antibodies
Antigens
Artificial immunity
B cells
Cell-mediated response
Cell surface marker
Complement
Endogenous
Exogenous
Humoral response
Immune response
Immunoglobulin
Inflammatory response
Interferon
Leukocytosis
Macrophage
Natural immunity
Nonspecific immunity
Nonspecific mechanisms
Opsonins
Passive immunity
Phagocytosis
Plasma
Specific immunity
Specific mechanisms
Susceptibility
T cells
Transient flora

II. Answer the following questions in the space provided.

1. List five biologic defense mechanisms of the body.

2. When antibodies are synthesized to the body in response to antigenic stimulation, it is called ________________.
3. The fluid portion of uncoagulated blood is called ________________.
4. Where is interferon produced? What is its function as a defense mechanism?

5. What are the three major physiologic responses that occur during the inflammatory process?

6. The ________________ is the control organ of the immune system.
7. What are the five cardinal symptoms of inflammation?

8. What is the difference between specific immunity and nonspecific immunity? Between active acquired immunity and passive acquired immunity?

9. What are two ways that a person acquires specific immunity?

III. For each situation below, indicate the type of immunity conferred by selecting the letter that corresponds with the description.

a. Natural active immunity
b. Artificial active immunity
c. Natural passive immunity
d. Artificial passive immunity

1. ______ A child recovering from chicken pox
2. ______ The transfer of maternal antibodies across the placenta to the neonate
3. ______ A child receiving a tetanus toxoid vaccine
4. ______ An adult receiving a gammaglobulin injection

IV. Match the duration of immunity with the type of immunity by selecting the appropriate letter below.

a. Lifetime
b. Temporary, lasting only a few months
c. Temporary, lasting only a few weeks
d. Several years, but requires a booster dose at specific intervals

1. ______ Natural passive immunity
2. ______ Natural active immunity
3. ______ Artificial active immunity
4. ______ Artificial passive immunity

V. For each statement below, write "T" if it refers to T cell lymphocytes or "B" if it refers to B cell lymphocytes:

1. ______ They are responsible for mediating cell-mediated immune responses.
2. ______ They are responsible for mediating humoral immune responses.
3. ______ They are known as thymus-dependent lymphocytes.
4. ______ They are produced by the thymus.
5. ______ They are referred to as thymus-independent lymphocytes.
6. ______ They are produced by the bursa.
7. ______ Responsible for immunity to viruses, cancer cells, and fungi.

8. _____ They produce antibodies (immunoglobulins) against the antigen.
9. _____ They do not destroy antigens by producing antibodies.
10. _____ They release lymphokines.

VI. Multiple choice

1. With inflammation, what response occurs after vasodilation?
   a. Vasoconstriction
   b. Fluid exudation
   c. Neutrophil migration
   d. Macrophage migration
2. The proteins in blood serum that have the ability to bind with antigens are called:
   a. Alpha-globulins
   b. Immunoglobulins
   c. Antigenic determinants
   d. Albumins
3. A systemic sign of severe inflammation includes:
   a. Hypertension
   b. Hypothermia
   c. Leukocytosis
   d. Phagocytosis
4. The cell-mediated (T cell) immune response has which of the following effects?
   a. Direct attack by activated lymphocytes
   b. Phagocytosis by macrophages
   c. Release of specific antigens
   d. Synthesis of antigen-specific immunoglobulins
5. The humoral (B cell) immune response has which of the following effects?
   a. Direct attack by activated lymphocytes
   b. Phagocytosis by macrophages
   c. Release of specific antigens
   d. Synthesis of antigen-specific immunoglobulins
6. Interferons are protective proteins produced by cells in response to:
   a. Drugs
   b. Virus
   c. Vaccine
   d. Immunoglobulins
7. Which are the most numerous and the most powerful of the phagocytic cells?
   a. Basophils
   b. Eosinophils
   c. Monocytes
   d. Neutrophils
8. An example of artificial active immunity is:
   a. Newborn
   b. Immunization
   c. Gamma-globulin
   d. Recovery from mumps
9. An inflammation that involves cellular or connective tissue is called:
   a. Emphysema
   b. Infection
   c. Cellutitis
   d. Connectivitis
10. Which class of immunoglobulins is predominant in adults and also provides the newborn with temporary immunity?
    a. IgD
    b. IgM
    c. IgA
    d. IgG
11. The reticuloendothelial system functions as a defense system by:
    a. Transporting blood and other substances to the site of injury
    b. Producing macrophages which do the final clean up at the site of injury
    c. Producing immunoglobulins
    d. Producing C-reactive proteins
12. Measurement of the C-reactive protein will:
    a. Provide information about the status of the reticuloendothelial system
    b. Help to determine the amount of protein needed in the diet of the infectious patient
    c. Help to identify the organisms causing the infection
    d. Provide information about the severity of the inflammation

VII. Test your assessment skills.

1. Assess the biologic defense mechanisms of a patient who has been injured in a car accident and brought to the emergency room. Be sure to include non specific mechanisms and specific mechanisms.

2. In a patient-teaching format, explain to a patient recovering from injuries the stages of the inflammatory response including how and when healing occurs.

SUGGESTED READINGS

Fidler, Sr, R: Deciphering diagnostic studies: complement assays Nursing 13:65-67, March 1983.
Defines complement and provides an overview of its function, its production, and its role in preventing infections. Outlines the purpose of complement assay tests, patient preparation, procedure, precautions, lab values, implications of results, post-test care, and interfering factors.

Jones, I: You can drive back infection if you know where to make your stand, Nursing 15:50-52, April 1985.
Provides a system-by-system guide to infection detection in the form of a chart. Reviews basic concept of colonization and describes things nurses can do to create barriers to infection. Identifies patients who are at risk for infection.

Taylor, DL: Immune response: physiology, signs, and symptoms, Nursing 14:52-54, May 1984.
Illustrations along with explanations about how the body recognizes and destroys antigens that threaten it and the clinical findings associated with these defense mechanisms.

Chapter 38

The Patient with Immunologic Problems

BRENDA GOODNER

CHAPTER OBJECTIVES

On completion of this chapter, the student should be able to:

- Identify the immune response in immunodeficiencies, gammopathies, hypersensitivities, and autoimmunities and give examples.
- Describe methods of immunosuppression and the care of the immunodeficient person.
- Describe the nature of AIDS and related care.
- Compare and contrast the four types of hypersensitivities.
- Describe the pathophysiologic bases of type I hypersensitivities and related interventions.
- Describe blood transfusion and tissue transplant reactions.

PREREQUISITE READING

Long-Phipps, Chapter 38, pp. 1353-1376.

SELF-ASSESSMENT ACTIVITIES

I. Define the following terms.

AIDS
Allergen
Allograft
Anaphylactic shock
Anergic
ARC
Autoimmune
Autotransfusion
Desensitization
Electrophoresis
ELISA
Gamma globulin
Hypersensitivity
Immunodeficiency
Sensitizing dose
Western blot test

II. Answer the following questions in the space provided.

1. What is gamma globulin?

2. Name the two tests used in diagnosing AIDS.

3. List five factors that influence hypersensitivity.

III. Fill in the chart by answering questions 1 through 3.

1. Place a check below each type of blood that can be received for each of the blood types listed in the chart at the right.
2. Based on the chart at the right, which blood type is the universal donor?
3. Based on the chart at the right, which blood type is the universal recipient?

Blood type	Blood type that can be received			
	A	B	AB	O
A				
B				
AB				
O				

IV. **A.** Complete the chart on problems related to blood transfusions.

Problems	Cause	Prevention
Bleeding		
Cardiac arrhythmias		
Hypocalcemia		
Hyperkalemia		
Transfusion hemosiderosis		

B. Complete the chart below on blood transfusion reactions.

Type of reaction	Symptoms	Occurrence	Action
Acute hemolytic			
Delayed hemolytic			
Allergic			
Febrile			
Graft versus host disease			
Noncardiac pulmonary edema			

C. Complete the chart below on allergy skin tests.

	Intradermal	Scratch	Patch	Conjunctival	Use
How is the test performed?					
What constitutes a positive reaction?					
When is the test read?					

V. Answer the following questions in the space provided.

1. List nine disorders at high risk of immunodeficiencies.

2. List the three effects of histamine.

3. What does the term Rh positive mean? Rh negative?

VI. Match the type of hypersensitivity reaction below with the appropriate description.

a. Anaphylactic **c.** Immune complex
b. Cytotoxic **d.** Cell-mediated

1. _____ Reactions of this type are mediated by the IgE class of immunoglobulins.
2. _____ Sensitivities can be transferred by lymphocyte exchange only.
3. _____ The primary pathologic effect involves release of histamines and kinins.
4. _____ Examples of this type include serum sickness, Arthus reaction, and glomerulonephritis.
5. _____ Examples of this type include hemolytic disease of the newborn (Rh) and transfusion reactions.
6. _____ Reactions of this type are mediated by T cells and macrophages.
7. _____ Examples of this type include systemic anaphylaxis, atopic allergies, and hay fever.
8. _____ Examples of this type include tuberculin reaction, skin graft rejection, and poison ivy.

VII. Multiple choice

1. To assess the status of an individual's immunoglobulins, which test would most likely be ordered?
   a. ELISA
   b. Electrophoresis
   c. CBC with differential count
   d. Bone marrow aspiration

2. The most important nursing goal while caring for an immunosuppressed patient is to:
   a. Help the patient accept the disease
   b. Prepare the patient to accept death
   c. Provide knowledge about the disease
   d. Protect the client from infection
3. The ELISA test:
   a. Screens blood or plasma for the presence of antibodies of the AIDS virus
   b. Can detect the AIDS virus
   c. Is used to diagnose AIDS
   d. Is used to establish a prognosis for the AIDS victim
4. A patient is admitted to your clinical unit with a diagnosis of AIDS. The patient has generalized weakness. No cough is present. Nursing care of this patient would include:
   a. Recapping needles securely before disposing
   b. Wearing gown and gloves when touching body secretions
   c. Using sterile disposable linens and equipment
   d. Assisting the patient to alter sexual habits
5. Which of the following best describes an inappropriate response to an antigen?
   a. T cell deficiency
   b. Gammopathy
   c. Hypersensitivity
   d. Autoimmunity

Jane Drone, age 4, is brought to the emergency room by her mother. Her mother states that Jane has been stung on the left arm by a bee. During the initial assessment, the nurse notices that Jane is sneezing and is scratching an edematous area on her left arm. Mrs. Drone tells the emergency department nurse that she believes Jane was stung for the first time in her life about 6 months ago.

6. The nurse realizes this sensitizing dose triggered the synthesis of antiallergic:
   a. IgA antibodies
   b. IgE antibodies
   c. IgG antibodies
   d. IgM antibodies
7. After a bee sting Jane's face becomes edematous and she begins to wheeze. Based on this assessment, the nurse would be prepared to administer:
   a. Aminophylline
   b. Benadryl
   c. Valium
   d. Epinephrine
8. Which of the following anaphylactic mediators is the most important in Jane's case?
   a. Serotonin
   b. Bradykinin
   c. Histamine
   d. Mast cells
9. Which of the following actions should Jane be taught to avoid anaphylactic reaction to a bee sting?
   a. Limit intake of sweets to reduce attraction of bees.
   b. Carry a dose of aminophylline with her at all times.
   c. Take precautionary actions when outdoors where bees are present.
   d. Wear a Medic-Alert tag that states she is allergic to histamine.

VIII. You are asked to teach a class on AIDS. Include the following information.

1. What is the causative agent of AIDS?

2. What is the mode of transmission?

3. What is the incubation period for the AIDS virus?

4. Who are persons at highest risk for AIDS?

5. Describe the test used to screen donated blood for AIDS.

6. List the primary immunologic pathophysiologic alterations in the individual with AIDS.

7. Give the names and list the manifestations of the two most common opportunistic infections that affect persons with AIDS.

8. What are the primary clinical manifestations of AIDS?

SUGGESTED READINGS

Anderson, D: AIDS: an update on what we now know, RN 49:49-56, Mar 1986.
Describes the transmission, incidence, prevention, and protective clothing to wear when caring for the AIDS victim.

Bennett, J: AIDS beyond the hospital: a two-part CE feature. What we know about AIDS, Am J Nurs 86:1015-1020, Sept 1986.
Current information on the causative organism (HIV), diagnosis, mode of transmission, and investigational drugs. Provides a chart showing the spectrum of HIV infection.

Dhundale, K: Home care for the AIDS patient: safety first, Nursing 16:34-36, Sept 1986.
Excellent article. Describes safety precautions that should be followed to protect the patient and the patient's caregivers, and family.

Hahn, AB, and others: Histamines and antihistamines, serotonin and antiserotonins. In Mosby's Pharmacology in nursing, St Louis, 1986, The CV Mosby Co.

Hahn, AB, and others: Replenishing fluids and electrolytes, blood components, and nutrients. In Mosby's Pharmacology in nursing, St Louis, 1986, The CV Mosby Co.

Kirkis, EJ and Ettorre, DM: Seven sticky problems (and their solutions) in blood transfusions, RN 46:59-62, April 1983.
Problems and solutions are described: incompatible solution is being run simultaneously through the infusion line; should blood be piggybacked through an IV line; wrong filter is being used to infuse blood; no instructions given about flow rate; improper and excessive handling of the bag of blood; blood administration set primed with wrong solution. Step-by-step instructions on how to set up a 'Y' set for blood administration. Outlines the dangers to watch for during a blood transfusion and appropriate actions.

Querin, JJ, and Stahl, LD: 12 simple sensible steps for successful blood transfusions, Nursing 13:34-44, Nov 1983.
Excellent article. Describes the procedure for administering blood and blood products. Explains nursing actions to prevent problems at each step of the transfusion procedure. Describes adverse reactions to blood transfusions, including cause, onset, symptoms, and nursing interventions. Provides a descriptive chart of all the blood products—their indications, equipment used, administration procedure, and special considerations.

Schietinger, H: A home care plan for AIDS patients, Am J Nurs 86:1021-1028, Sept 1986.
Describes chronic symptoms of HIV infections, the impact of the diagnosis, how to intervene with common chronic problems experienced by AIDS patients. A list of AIDS resources throughout the US is provided.

The Committee on Transfusion Practices: The latest protocols for blood transfusion, Nursing 16:34-41, Oct 1986.
Explains the following nursing protocols: identifying the patient, obtaining the blood sample for typing and crossmatching, labeling the sample, obtaining blood components from the blood bank, identifying the patient and blood component before transfusion, adding saline to blood components, using blood filters, maintaining the proper infusion rate, using blood warmers, administering irradiated blood components, and detecting and responding to hemolytic transfusion reactions.

Chapter 39

The Patient with Dermatologic Problems

BRENDA GOODNER

CHAPTER OBJECTIVES

On completion of this chapter, the student should be able to:

- Describe the psychologic effect of skin disorders.
- Differentiate skin inflammations resulting from bacteria, viruses, fungi, and parasites and describe appropriate therapy.
- Describe methods of applying medications to the skin.
- Describe measures for relief of pruritus.
- Differentiate between contact and atopic dermatitis and methods of prevention.
- Describe the pathophysiology of psoriasis and therapeutic measures.
- Describe the different types of skin tumors and surgical interventions.
- Describe the different types of grafts and measures to promote healing.
- Identify different types of cosmetic surgeries.

PREREQUISITE READING

Long-Phipps, Chapter 39, pp. 1377-1406.

SELF-ASSESSMENT ACTIVITIES

I. Define the following terms.

Autograft
Candidiasis
Cellulitis
Conduction
Convection
Dermatitis
Dermis
Epidermis
Evaporation
Heterograft
Homograft
Kaposi's sarcoma
Keloids
Keratosis
Liposuction
Melanoma
Psoriasis
Rhinoplasty
Rhytidoplasty
Scabies
Shingles
Subcutaneous tissue
Tinea capitis
Tinea corporis
Tinea cruris
Tinea pedis

II. Answer the following questions in the space provided.

1. List five functions of the skin.

2. The drug of choice for athlete's foot is ________________.
3. List the four most common parasitic infections.

4. The malignant disorder commonly seen in AIDS patients is ________________.

5. The skin graft that covers the epidermis and all of the dermis is the ________________ graft.
6. Describe a free-flap graft.

III. Complete the following chart on infections of the skin.

Infections	Etiology	Clinical manifestations	Medical management	Nursing management
Folliculitis				
Furuncles				
Carbuncles				
Cellulitis				
Warts				
Herpes simplex				
Herpetic whitlow				
Herpes zoster				

IV. Complete the following reference chart on parasitic and fungal infestations of the skin.

Infestation	Etiology	Clinical manifestations	Medical management	Nursing management
Pediculosis	Head louse Body louse Pubic louse			
Scabies	Sarcoptes Scabili (female itch mite)	Wavy, brownish, threadlike lines, usually on hands	Treatment of patient and all family with:	Primarily teaching 1. 2. 3. 4.
Candidiasis	*Candida albicans* Thrush			
Tinea capitis				
Tinea corporis				
Tinea cruris				
Tinea pedis				

V. Fill in the following information about pruritis.

1. Etiology

2. Pathophysiology

3. Clinical manifestations

4. Relief of the itch-scratch cycle

VI. Multiple choice

1. The most important function of the skin is to:
   a. Protect the underlying tissue from the outer environment
   b. Maintain temperature
   c. Maintain circulation
   d. Remove body water
2. Dressings are sometimes used to debride wounds or ulcerations. The moist gauze is allowed to dry over a lesion and then be removed. Which of the following dressings is used for this purpose?
   a. Open wet dressing
   b. Closed wet dressing
   c. Wet-to-wet dressing
   d. Wet-to-dry dressing
3. Which of the following actions is most effective when applying dermatologic wet dressings?
   a. Use sterile technique
   b. Apply at cold temperatures
   c. Apply continuously for 24 hours
   d. Apply damp but not dripping
4. The most common procedure used in plastic surgery is grafting. The best results are obtained from:
   a. Autografts
   b. Homografts
   c. Heterograft
   d. Xenograft
5. Free full-thickness grafts are used mainly to cover small areas because:
   a. The blood supply cannot become extablished quickly
   b. Regeneration of skin at the donor site is impossible
   c. Infection is prone to develop
   d. Pedicle grafts predispose to gangrene
6. Katie Andrews, age 16, will undergo a rhinoplasty. While talking to her in a patient teaching session, the nurse tells her that to decrease swelling:
   a. "We will be putting heating pads over your face."
   b. "We will be putting ice bags on your face."
   c. "You will be positioned sitting straight up."
   d. "You will not be allowed much pain medication."
7. Katie asks, "How long will it be before I can see how the surgery will alter my appearance?" The correct answer is:
   a. "It will take several weeks to see final results."
   b. "When the bandages come off you will be able to tell."
   c. "When the swelling goes down you will see results."
   d. "Do not expect too much. There are not always changes."
8. Which of the following skin tumors is most highly malignant?
   a. Actinic keratoses
   b. Melanoma
   c. Basal cell carcinoma
   d. Squamous cell carcinoma
9. A deep infection around a hair follicle is termed a:
   a. Carbuncle
   b. Cellulitis
   c. Folliculitis
   d. Furuncle
10. Teaching for the person with athlete's foot should include:
    a. Avoid walking barefoot in gyms
    b. Wash feet after swimming in pool
    c. Wear white socks to keep feet clean
    d. Go barefoot often and keep feet dry
11. Herpes zoster, or shingles, is a disease process of clusters of small vesicles that follow the pathway of sensory nerves. The rash can occur on the back, face, and scalp. The major problem with herpes zoster is:
    a. Highly contagious
    b. Pain and itching
    c. Difficult to heal
    d. No effective therapy
12. Patient teaching with teenagers who take Accutane for acne must include which important side effect?
    a. Brittle hair
    b. Dry lips
    c. Low libido
    d. Birth defects
13. If tetracycline is taken for treatment of acne, what precaution should the nurse advise the patient to take?
    a. Use birth control pills
    b. Avoid high-fat foods
    c. Do not take other drugs
    d. Avoid direct sunlight

VII. Match the following.

1. _____ Callus	**a.** malignant tumor over hairy areas
2. _____ Leukoplakia	**b.** Malignant tumor of epidermis
3. _____ Basal cell carcinoma	**c.** Thick, horny skin layer
4. _____ Squamous cell carcinoma	**d.** Thick, white patch
5. _____ Malignant melanoma	**e.** Serious skin cancer

VIII. Write a nursing care plan for the following.

1. A patient with a fungal inflammation.

2. A patient with a skin graft.

SUGGESTED READINGS

Berliner, H: Aging skin: part two, Am J Nurs 86:1259-1261, Nov 1986.
Twelve photographs accompany short explanations of common skin problems of aging skin, blood lesions, and skin carcinoma.

Perry, A, and Potter, B: Fundamentals of nursing, St Louis, 1985, The CV Mosby Co.
Review and study of personal hygiene, chapters on hair and skin care, application of heat and cold, and bandaging.

Chapter 40

The Patient with Burns

BRENDA GOODNER
MARY S. NICHOLS

CHAPTER OBJECTIVES

On completion of this chapter, the student should be able to:

- Differentiate between partial-thickness and full-thickness burns.
- Describe the pathophysiologic changes that occur during the three stages following major burns.
- Describe the emergency care for major burns and the initial inpatient therapy.
- Describe interventions for replacing body fluids, preventing infection, promoting nutrition and mobility, and providing emotional support.
- Identify teaching needs of the patient with burns.

PREREQUISITE READING

Long-Phipps, Chapter 40, pp. 1407-1440.

SELF-ASSESSMENT ACTIVITIES

I. Define the following terms.

Autograft	Homograft	Split-thickness graft
Deep partial-thickness burn	Hyperkalemia	Stamping
Eschar	Jobst garment	Superficial partial-thickness burn
Full-thickness burn	Meshing	
Heterograft	Partial-thickness burn	

II. Complete the following.

1. The three periods of treatment for a seriously burned patient are:

2. The ____________________ is used to determine the percentage of the body surface burned.
3. The two age groups with the highest mortality rate are:

4. Name five factors which help determine the severity of the burn:

5. List one advantage of each method of burn wound care:
   a. Open method: ____________________
   b. Semi-open method: ____________________
   c. Closed method: ____________________

6. A major goal in discharge teaching is to prevent excessive scar formation by teaching the patient proper ______________________, ______________________, and ______________________.
7. The burn victim's need for ______________________ is increased by two to four times the amount required before injury.
8. Temporary skin grafts now in use are: (a) ______________________ and (b) ______________________.
9. Therapeutic positioning, splints, and exercises for burn patients are aimed at the prevention or correction of ______________________.
10. List six topical medications used in burn therapy.

III. Multiple choice

1. Ann Stewart was conducting an experiment in the chemistry lab at Riverview High School which resulted in an explosion and burns to her hands and arms. The preferred first aid treatment would be:
   a. Immediately place an ice pack on the burned area.
   b. Cover the burns with petroleum jelly or butter.
   c. Ascertain the purpose of the experiment she was conducting.
   d. Remove the chemical agent from her hands and arms by flushing with water.
2. The primary effects seen in a severe burn, when fluid shifts from the vascular compartment into the interstitial spaces, are all *except:*
   a. Increased urinary output
   b. Decreased blood pressure
   c. Edema
   d. Increased hematocrit
3. Which is *not* likely to occur during the diuretic stage?
   a. Diuresis
   b. Fluid overload
   c. Hyperkalemia
   d. Metabolic acidosis
4. When calculating fluid replacement therapy the time will be calculated from:
   a. An estimate of the length of expected hospital stay
   b. The time patient is seen in the emergency room
   c. The time of the injury
   d. The time of patient's first voiding
5. Which method of pain relief is *not* recommended for extensive burns?
   a. Gentle and minimal handling.
   b. Application of dressings that exclude air
   c. Ice packs applied directly to burn area
   d. Cool compresses applied to burn site while keeping victim warm
6. Full-thickness burns:
   a. Destroy the dermis and epidermis but not the nerve endings
   b. May result from complications of a deep partial-thickness burn
   c. Are extremely painful but never require skin grafting
   d. Are the same as first degree burns
7. All of the following biochemical imbalances occur with extensive severe burns during the first 48 to 72 hours *except:*
   a. Hyperkalemia
   b. Hypoprotienemia
   c. Hypernatremia
   d. Metabolic acidosis

8. Which is the drug of choice for pain relief for burn victims?
   a. Morphine sulfate drip
   b. Morphine injected subcutaneously
   c. Codeine
   d. Aspirin or Tylenol
9. When hypovolemic shock occurs:
   a. There is an increase in blood pressure and inadequate blood flow through the kidneys.
   b. There is a slight drop in blood pressure and inadequate blood flow through the kidneys.
   c. There is a tremendous drop in blood pressure and inadequate blood flow through the kidneys.
   d. There is a drop in blood pressure and adequate blood flow through the kidneys.
10. Partial-thickness burns:
    a. Are not painful as only the epidermis is affected
    b. Will not heal because the epithelial cells have been destroyed
    c. Involve a part of the epidermis and dermis
    d. Usually require skin grafting
11. The hypovolemic stage:
    a. Begins 48 to 72 hours after the burn injury
    b. Is characterized by a rapid shift of fluid from the interstitial spaces into the vascular compartments
    c. Begins at the time of the burn injury and lasts about ten days
    d. Is characterized by a rapid shift of fluid from the vascular compartments into the interstitial spaces

The doctor explains to Ron Hayes that a skin graft will be required for both his thighs. To provide permanent coverage, skin will be taken from Ron's back and placed on his thighs.

12. This type of skin graft is called:
    a. Homograft
    b. Zenograft
    c. Heterograft
    d. Autograft
13. The doctor further explains that the strip of skin taken from Ron's back will be fed into an instrument which perforates the sheet of skin with tiny slits. The skin grafting method is called:
    a. Meshing
    b. Stamping
    c. Shredding
    d. Molding

Active range of motion exercises are prescribed for Ron. When you enter his room to have him perform the exercises that were planned by the physical therapist, he states, "I just can't do those exercises. It's too painful. Can't I wait until my burns have healed?"

14. Which response by the nurse would be most appropriate?
    a. "No. We can't wait. The doctor has ordered the exercises and you must do them."
    b. "You're going to have to do them or you'll never be able to walk or use your arms again."
    c. "We'll arrange for you to do the exercises after you have had your pain medication."
    d. "I'll talk with the doctor to have the exercises postponed until your burns have had time to heal."
15. Ron Hayes undergoes a skin graft. Postoperatively, he returns to the unit with a pressure dressing over his thighs. The physician has also prescribed a heat lamp to the donor site. The primary purpose of the heat lamp is to:
    a. Keep Ron warm
    b. Aid in drying the site
    c. Enhance visibility of the site
    d. Kill bacteria

16. The nurse writes the following order on Ron's care plan: Observe for lactose intolerance. The primary symptoms of a lactose intolerance are all *except:*
   a. Constipation
   b. Diarrhea
   c. Flatulence
   d. Bloating
17. The burn victim is started on exercises for prevention and correction contractures:
   a. On admission to the hospital
   b. After the pain is gone
   c. As soon as his/her condition is stable
   d. 48 hours after the time of injury

CASE STUDY

Jason Rogers, age 14, and his friend Rob were camping out in Jason's backyard. Jason had spilled some lighter fluid on his pants while getting the grill and charcoal from the garage. When he struck the match to light the charcoal, his pants ignited immediately. He began running wildly and screaming, "Help!" Rob ran into the house to get Jason's mother.

An ambulance was called and Jason was transported to the emergency room. When the doctor asked Mrs. Rogers when Jason's last tetanus shot was she replied, "I don't know. It was such a long time ago."

Jason had sustained burns over the areas shaded in the illustration below. Use this illustration to answer the questions on p. 261.

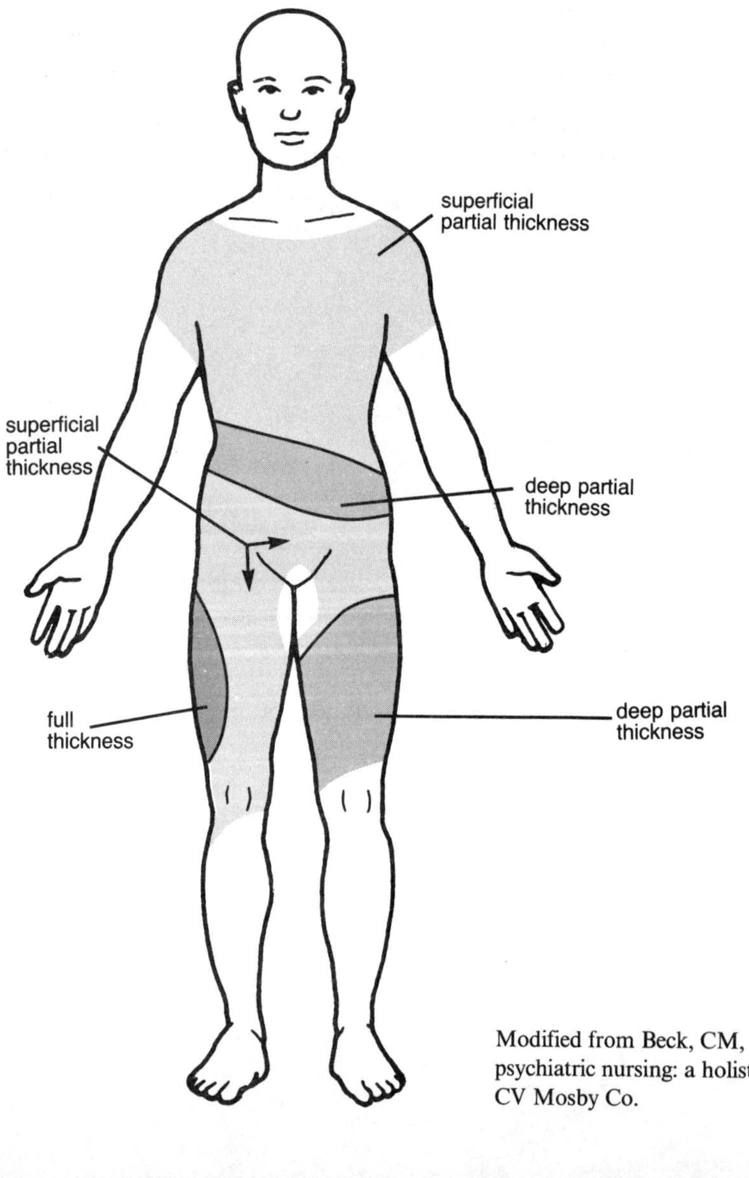

Modified from Beck, CM, Rawlins, RP and Williams SR: Mental health-psychiatric nursing: a holistic life-cycle approach, ed 2, St Louis, 1987, The CV Mosby Co.

1. Which areas of Jason's burns would form blisters?

2. Which areas of Jason's burns would not be painful? Why?

3. What form of tetanus immunization will Jason be given since his prior tetanus immunization is unknown?

SUGGESTED READINGS

Hurt, RA: More than skin deep: guidelines on caring for the burn patient, Nursing 15:52-57, June 1985.
The author describes the problems that occur during the resuscitation phase, the acute care phase, and the home care phase and interventions to resolve and/or prevention problems.

Johnson, CL and Cain, VJ: The rehab guide, Am J Nurs 85:48-50, Jan 1985.
The authors provide a chart with explanations on how to exercise newly burned areas of each body part.

Rich, J: Lightning injury, Nursing 16:25, June 1986.
The author outlines the decision-making process when intervening at the scene of a lightning injury, and describes priorities in treatment.

Robertson, K, and others: Burn care: for CE credit: the crucial days, Am J Nurs 85:29-45, Jan 1985.
Excellent article. Describes on-site treatment of each type of burn injury, emergency department priorities, how to estimate the size and depth of a burn, wound care, fluid needs, nutritional support, rehabilitation needs, and psychosocial care during each phase. Great pictures.

Rosequist, CC, and Shepp, PH: The nutrition factor, Am J Nurs 85:45-47, Jan 1985.
Provides a formulary of several methods on how to calculate nutritional needs, describes parameters of a nutritional assessment, and outlines nutritional needs of the burn victim during each phase.

UNIT XI Emergent and Critical Care

Chapter 41

Problems Encountered in Emergencies and Disasters

BRENDA GOODNER

CHAPTER OBJECTIVES

On completion of this chapter, the student should be able to:

- Describe preventive methods for accidents.
- Describe the nature of delivery of emergency care.
- Describe parameters of assessment of the injured or unconscious person.
- Identify principles of general management and specific care for accidental injuries or sudden illness (cardiac arrest, MI, near drowning, electrical injuries, poisoning, excess heat or cold, radiation, wounds, and fractures).
- Discuss the nature of rape and appropriate interventions.
- Describe the effects of disasters and appropriate roles of the nurse during disasters.

PREREQUISITE READING

Long-Phipps, Chapter 41, pp. 1443-1469.

SELF-ASSESSMENT ACTIVITIES

I. Define the following terms.

Abrasion
Asphyxia
Cardiopulmonary resuscitation (CPR)
Contusion
Disaster
Dislocation
Dry drowning
Flail chest
Fracture
Frostbite
Good Samaritan laws
Head-to-toe assessment
Heat exhaustion
Heat stroke
Heimlich abdominal thrust maneuver
Hemothorax
Hypothermia
Hypoxia
Incision
Laceration
Near-drowning
Pneumothorax
Priority assessment
Puncture
Secondary drowning
Shock
Stab
Tension pneumothorax
Triage
Wet drowning

II. Complete the chart on poisons below.

Type of poison	Interventions
Inhaled poison: carbon monoxide	
Contact insecticides	
Ingested poison: lye	
Ingested poison: drugs	
Insect stings: wasps and bees	
Tick bites	

III. Complete the chart on extreme exposure to heat and cold.

General reactions	Cause	Signs and symptoms	Interventions
Heat cramps			
Heat exhaustion			
Heat stroke			
Frostbite			

IV. Multiple choice

While driving along the highway late one evening, you discover an overturned automobile. The driver is still in the automobile with his head leaning against the steering wheel.

1. Which of the following actions would be most important?
   a. Go for more help immediately
   b. Check the level of consciousness and breathing
   c. Look for identification of the victim
   d. Check the victim for adequate circulation
2. You would conclude that the victim is in shock if which of the following are found?
   a. Cool, clammy skin, rapid respirations
   b. Slow pulse
   c. Slow respirations
   d. Flushed color
3. Initial intervention for external bleeding would involve:
   a. Elevation of the affected part above the level of the heart
   b. Direct pressure over the bleeding vessel
   c. Application of ice
   d. Application of a tourniquet
4. Tetanus can be prevented by:
   a. Protective isolation
   b. Thorough handwashing
   c. Immunization
   d. Thorough cooking of foods
5. Clinical manifestations of tetanus include:
   a. Headaches and dizziness
   b. Nausea and vomiting
   c. Diarrhea and abdominal cramps
   d. Muscle rigidity and spasms
6. Initial treatment for an open pneumothorax would include:
   a. Keeping the victim flat and supine
   b. Insertion of a chest tube
   c. Covering with a nonporous material
   d. Administration of oxygen
7. A patient is diagnosed as having flail chest. You would expect to find:
   a. Symmetrical rise and fall of the chest with inspiration and expiration
   b. Rise of the affected side with inspiration and fall of the unaffected side
   c. No chest movement at all
   d. Fall of the affected side with inspiration when the unaffected side rises
8. In the management of a fracture, which of the following would be contraindicated?
   a. Applying splints to include joint above and below the fracture
   b. Straightening deformities of a joint before splinting
   c. Applying gentle traction to straighten severe angulation when the shaft of a bone is fractured
   d. Splinting the fracture in the position found
9. A mother brings her six-year-old son to the emergency room and says frantically, "I think my son has just taken all of my Valium tablets. He probably thought they were his new vitamins." Which data are most important for the nurse to obtain?
   a. Where the mother keeps the Valium tablets
   b. The name of the doctor who prescribed the Valium tablets
   c. The number of Valium tablets in the bottle and the dosage
   d. The color and name brand of the child's vitamins

10. A patient who has suffered a concussion will have:
    a. Equal pupils
    b. Unequal pupils
    c. Nystagmus
    d. Blank stare
11. Electrical burns can cause multiple injuries. The injury most likely to cause death is:
    a. Depression of respirations
    b. Internal tissue damage
    c. Multiple bone fractures
    d. Ventricular fibrillation
12. What is the first action to be taken when a person is injured?
    a. Rapidly assess for priority data
    b. Determine lifesaving interventions
    c. Transport to nearest medical facility
    d. Prepare to carry out CPR immediately
13. What is the legal aspect on which nurses would be held liable under law when giving emergency care?
    a. Complications arising from injuries
    b. Injury resulting from negligence
    c. Not stopping at scene of accident
    d. Temporarily functioning as a physician
14. What is the first priority in assessment of an injured person?
    a. Fractures
    b. Level of consciousness
    c. Hemorrhage
    d. Airway patency

V. Test your skill at assessment and intervention.

Situation	Assessment	Interventions
1. You and another swimmer dive into a swimming pool to rescue a near-drowning teenager. When the victim is pulled onto the pool deck, you discover that he is not breathing.		
2. While riding in a city bus, an elderly male sitting next to you suddenly becomes diaphoretic, complaining of severe, radiating chest pain, and difficulty breathing. He is dressed in a business suit. You suspect that the person is experiencing an MI.		
3. While climbing the stairs to your apartment, you see an elderly female lying on the floor. Particles of food are around her mouth and her right hand is lying on her chest below her neck. She is unconscious. You suspect obstructed airway.		
4. While dining in a cafe, a middle-aged male suddenly stands up grasping his throat and motioning with his lips "Help, Help." You suspect obstructed airway.		

SUGGESTED READINGS

Blauer, RE: Dealing with near-drownings, RN 48:41-42, May 1985.

Describes the initial steps in the treatment of an unconscious near-drowning victim at the scene and in the emergency department of the hospital.

DiNitto, D, et al: After rape: who should examine rape survivors?, Am J Nurs 86:538-540, May 1986.

Describes the rape crisis program used in Hillsborough County, Florida, the role of the nurses in the program, pros and cons of having nurse rape examiners, components of the rape kit exam, and cost of the examination and sources of financial assistance.

Jones, S: New IV catheters that can do it all, RN 48:20-23, Feb 1985.

Describes the types of triple-lumen catheters, what to do before and after insertion, complications and their prevention, and how to dispose of the catheters.

King, RC and Giles, J: Dealing with insect bites, RN 47:53-55, May 1984.

Excellent article. Describes reactions to and care of benign insect bites, tick bites, stings from the hymenoptera order of insects (wasp, bees), and bites from spiders and scorpions.

Kuhn, PJ: What kind of food poisoning is it?, RN 48:39-41, June 1985.

Identifies causes of food poisoning, tells how to evaluate bacterial food poisoning, and describes manifestations and treatment.

LaVoy, K: Dealing with hypothermia and frostbite, RN 48:53-56, Jan 1985.

Excellent article. Describes how to spot individuals with hypothermia and how to treat them in the field and in the emergency department.

Niemczura, J: Eight rules to remember when caring for a Swan-Ganz catheter, Nursing 15:38-41, March 1985.

Explains each of the following eight rules: learn why the patient has the Swan-Ganz catheter; take readings during a fluid challenge or other therapeutic maneuver and always check with the doctor when the PCWP goes above 20 mm Hg or deviates dramatically from prevailing trends; know benefits, adverse reactions, and nursing implications for drugs that you begin to monitor with the Swan-Ganz catheter; aim at improving cardiac output not blood pressure; maximize preload and minimize afterload; don't try to manipulate preload, contractility, and afterload all at once; catheter; learn more about your hospital's policies for the use of a Swanz-Ganz catheter.

Scordo, K: Hemodynamic monitoring: Learning to read the waves, Nursing 15:40-42, July 1985.

Provides an explanation of insertion of a balloon-tipped pulmonary artery catheter and what type of waveforms to anticipate as the catheter is threaded through the heart chambers and finally into the pulmonary artery. Gives tips on taking PAWP and how to interpret the waveforms.

Sebilia, AJ: When was your last tetanus shot? RN 47:18-24, Aug 1984.

Excellent article. Through a case study, the author describes manifestations of tetanus, emergency treatments and nursing care, who's at risk of tetanus, and prevention.

Chapter 42

Care of the Patient in a Critical Care Unit

BRENDA GOODNER

CHAPTER OBJECTIVES

On completion of this chapter, the student should be able to:

- Describe the physical and psychologic environment of critical care units.
- Identify the types of data needed for the care of critically ill patients.
- Describe interventions to alleviate physiologic stressors (respiratory, cardiovascular, neurologic, renal, gastrointestinal, musculoskeletal/integumentary) which are specific to the critical care setting.
- Describe interventions to alleviate and prevent psychologic stressors for both the patient and the nurse.

PREREQUISITE READING

Long-Phipps, Chapter 42, pp. 1471-1491.

SELF-ASSESSMENT ACTIVITIES

I. Define the following terms.

Adult respiratory distress syndrome (ARDS)
Baseline assessment
Central venous pressure (CVP)
Continuous arteriovenous hemofiltration (CAVH)
Hemodialysis
Hemodynamic monitoring
Intraarterial monitoring
Intracranial pressure (ICP)
Invasive techniques
Peritoneal dialysis
Positive-end expiratory pressure (PEEP)
Pulmonary capillary wedge pressure (PCWP)
Swan-Ganz catheter
Total parenteral nutrition (TPN)

II. Answer the following questions:

1. What is a baseline assessment? What is the purpose of this assessment?

2. The primary intervention for ARDS is ____________________.
3. List seven complications of intraarterial monitoring.

4. List seven potential complications of Swan-Ganz monitoring.

5. Signs and symptoms of pulmonary embolism are:

6. What does PEEP do?

7. List 11 nursing interventions to prevent increased ICP in a critically ill patient.

8. Compare and differentiate among hemodialysis, peritoneal dialysis, and continous arteriovenous hemofiltration.

9. What drug is administered for stress ulcers in the ICU patient?

III. Match the terms below with the appropriate formula.

a. Cardiac output
b. Cardiac index
c. Stroke volume
d. Stroke index
e. Mean arterial pressure
f. Pulmonary vascular resistance
g. Systemic vascular resistance

1. _____ $\dfrac{\text{MAP} - \text{CVP} \times 80}{\text{cardiac output}}$

2. _____ $\dfrac{\text{stroke volume}}{\text{body surface area}}$

3. _____ heart rate $\times$ stroke volume

4. _____ $\dfrac{\text{cardiac output}}{\text{heart rate}}$

5. _____ $\dfrac{\text{mean PAP} - \text{mean PCWP}}{\text{cardiac output}}$

6. _____ 2/3 diastolic + 1/3 systolic

7. _____ $\dfrac{\text{cardiac output}}{\text{body surface area}}$

IV. Complete the following chart after studying Table 42-3 on p. 1483 of the text.

Drug	Method of administration	Clinical purpose
Atropine sulfate		
Bretylium tosylate (Bretylol)		
Calcium chloride		
Digoxin (Lanoxin)		
Dopamine hydrochloride (Intropin)		
Dobutamine hydrochloride (Dobutrex)		
Epinephrine hydrochloride (Adrenalin)		
Isoproterenol hydrochloride (Isuprel)		
Lidocaine hydrochloride (Xylocaine)		
Morphine sulfate		
Nitroglycerin (Nitro-Bid IV)		
Nitroprusside sodium (Nipride)		
Norepinephrine (Levarterenol, Levophed)		
Propranolol (Inderal)		
Sodium bicarbonate		
Verapamil (Calan, Isoptin)		

V. Multiple choice

1. The pulmonary artery (Swan-Ganz) catheter:
   a. Is floated through the left side of the heart
   b. Has a balloon at the distal tip that lies in the pulmonary artery
   c. Is inserted into the aorta through the superior vena cava
   d. Is used to measure pressure within the alveoli
2. Which of the following hemodynamic monitoring devices can be used to obtain cardiac output measurements?
   a. Pulmonary artery catheter (Swan-Ganz)
   b. Intraarterial catheter
   c. Cardiac monitor
   d. Intracranial monitoring
3. To maintain patency of the intraarterial catheter, it should be flushed:
   a. Once per shift
   b. Once every hour
   c. Once a day
   d. Only when ordered by the physician
4. From which of the following hemodynamic monitoring devices can samples be taken for arterial blood gas analysis?
   a. Intraarterial catheter
   b. Swanz-Ganz catheter
   c. Both
   d. Neither
5. Adult respiratory distress syndrome may also be referred to as:
   a. Chronic respiratory failure
   b. Acute respiratory failure
   c. Da Nang lung
   d. Shock lung
6. The development of ARDS is characterized by which of the following sets of symptoms?
   a. Hypoxemia, increased work of breathing, and grunting respirations
   b. Bradypnea, confusion, and hypotension
   c. Increased pulmonary secretions and respiratory acidosis
   d. White pulmonary infiltrates on x-ray and low pCO_2
7. The first step in management of critically ill patients involves:
   a. Establishing a data base
   b. Identifying real and potential problems
   c. Delineating priorities
   d. Defining outcome criteria
8. During the initial admission of the patient to the ICU, emphasis is placed on:
   a. Interviewing the family members so that crucial facts about the patient can be assessed
   b. Alleviating physiologic threats to survival
   c. Developing rapport with the family
   d. Orienting the patient to the ICU environment
9. The normal range for cardiac output is:
   a. 2.5-4.0 $l/min/m^2$
   b. 35-70 $ml/beats/m^2$
   c. 4.0-8.0 l/min
   d. 70-90 l/beats/min
10. The first line intervention in severe cardiovascular disorders is:
    a. Drug therapy
    b. Cardiopulmonary resuscitation
    c. Hemodynamic monitoring
    d. Permanent pacemaker

11. Planning for the cardiac patient in the ICU emphasizes:
    a. Systemic circulation
    b. Decreasing blood pressure, pulse
    c. Decreasing myocardial workload
    d. Increasing physical exertion
12. When ICP is being monitored via intraventricular catheter, what is the top priority nursing intervention?
    a. Constant monitoring of ICP waveform
    b. Meticulous care to prevent infection
    c. Removal of CSF if ICP increases
    d. Monitor for cardiac dysrhythmias
13. The ICU nurse observes the patient in renal failure for ECG changes, Kussmaul breathing, and decreased LOC. This assessment is monitoring for:
    a. Metabolic acidosis
    b. Metabolic alkalosis
    c. Electrolyte imbalance
    d. Cardiac complications
14. The most common gastrointestinal problem seen in the ICU is:
    a. Evisceration
    b. Peritonitis
    c. GI bleeding
    d. Infections
15. Most of the documenting of ongoing data in the ICU is done by:
    a. Nurse's notes
    b. SOAP notes
    c. Flow sheets
    d. Problem-oriented records

VI. Test your assessment and intervention skills. For each of the stressors for ICU patients listed below write the appropriate nursing intervention for prevention and alleviation.

1. Unfamiliar environment and faces

2. High noise and light levels

3. Sensory deprivation or overload

4. Interruption of sleep/wake cycles

5. Inaccessibility of family and friends

6. Lack of information and understanding of prognosis and care plan

7. Lack of information and understanding of policies and procedures

8. Anticipation of painful interventions

9. Confusion and disorientation related to physiologic factors

10. Impaired communication related to intubation

11. Fear related to diagnosis

12. Fear of death

SUGGESTED READINGS

LeMay, CM: How we prep patients for the ICU, RN 49:44-45, May 1986.
The author describes how she used an album full of photos of the ICU and an audiocassette tape to explain the pictures to tell patients what to expect during their stay in ICU.
Wall, C: Making life bearable for your chronic ICU patients, RN 48:61-68, May 1985.
Five steps to making the ICU less stressful are explained: relaxation techniques, use of recreation, use of physical therapy, use of social services, and how to ease the transfer from the ICU.

Answer Key

Chapter 1

	Answer	Page reference
II.	1. a	5
	2. c	4
	3. d	7
	4. a	7
	5. d	7
	6. d	6
	7. d	6, 7
	8. a	7
	9. b	8
	10. a	9

Chapter 2

	Answer	Page reference
III.	1. d	13
	2. b	14
	3. b	15, 19
	4. c	16
	5. c	15
	6. a	16
	7. d	18-20
	8. a	21

	Answer	Answer
IV.	1. O	6. O
	2. S	7. S
	3. S	8. S
	4. O	9. O
	5. O	10. S
VI.	1. I	3. I
	2. C	4. I

Chapter 3

	Answer	Page reference
II.	1. *See box.*	26-27
	2. *See text.*	27
	3. *See text.*	27
	4. *See text.*	29
	5. *See box.*	26
	6. *See box.*	43
III.	1. d	33
	2. g	33
	3. f	33
	4. c	33
	5. e	33
	6. a	33
	7. b	33

Chapter 3 (cont'd)

	Answer	Page reference
IV.	1. d	31
	2. a	27
	3. b	27
	4. c	30
	5. c	31
	6. d	34
	7. a	35
	8. b	36
	9. c	41
	10. a	42

Chapter 4

	Answer	Page reference
II.	1. d	46
	2. b	46
	3. a	46
	4. c	46
	5. d	48
	6. b	49
	7. c	49
	8. b	49
	9. a	49
	10. d	49
	11. d	49
	12. b	49
	13. b	53
	14. b	53
	15. d	48
	16. b	51
	17. d	53

Chapter 5

	Answer	Page reference
II.	1. Leaving the family of origin; establishing a new home base; choosing a life-style; developing sexual bonding; reexamining commitments; choosing a vocation.	61
	2. Adjusting to declining physical strength and health; accepting reorganized family patterns; adjusting to retirement and change in financial status; to a new pattern of social and civic responsibilities; establishing affiliation with one's group; maintaining satisfactory living arrangements; developing point of view about death.	67
	3. *See text.*	60-62
	4. *See text.*	63-65

	Answer	Page reference
III.	1. c	63
	2. d	60
	3. b	67
	4. c	70
	5. c	70

Chapter 5 (cont'd)

	Answer	Page reference
III.	6. b	
	7. a	73
	8. d	70
	9. d	70
	10. c	62
	11. d	67
	12. c	66
	13. a	72-73
	14. d	60
	15. b	60
	16. d	72
IV.	*See chart*	66

Chapter 6

	Answer	Page reference
V.	1. c	83
	2. d	84
	3. b	79
	4. c	86
	5. b	87
	6. a	88
	7. d	91
	8. d	91
	9. c	91
	10. b	91
	11. d	91
	12. c	92
	13. a	92
	14. b	92
	15. c	92

Chapter 7

	Answer	Page reference
II.	1. c	100
	2. d	101
	3. d	101
	4. b	113
	5. d	105
	6. b	103
	7. a	104
	8. d	110
III.	1. c	110
	2. b	110
	3. d, a	110
	4. g	109
	5. h	104
	6. i	113
	7. e, f	102

Chapter 8

	Answer	Page reference
VI.	1. c	122
	2. d	122
	3. a	122
	4. a	123
	5. c	136
	6. d	129
	7. b	132
	8. b	134
	9. c	132, 133
	10. d	133
	11. b	123, 124
	12. a	128
	13. a	129
	14. d	129
	15. c	126, 127
	16. b	122, 123
VII.	1. a	122
	2. c	123
	3. d	122
	4. a	122
	5. c	122
	6. b	123
	7. d	122
	8. b	123
	9. a	122
	10. d	122
	11. c	123
IX.	1. b	
	2. b	128
	3. d	131
	4. a	140
	5. b	122
	6. a	122
	7. c	
	8. d	129
	9. b	126
	10. b	129
	11. a	131
	12. a	126, 124
	13. b	127
	14. d	131, 132

Chapter 9

	Answer	Page reference
I.	1. c	146
	2. a	146
	3. d	146-147
	4. b	147

Chapter 9 (cont'd)

	Answer	Page reference
III.	1. d	144
	2. a	144
	3. b	144
	4. a	144
	5. d	147
	6. c	144
	7. d	144
	8. d	147
	9. a	144
	10. b	144
	11. d	145
	12. d	145
	13. b	146
	14. a	146
	15. d	146
	16. c	148, 155
	17. c	149
	18. a	149
	19. b	151
	20. c	151
	21. b	148
	22. c	162
	23. d	163
	24. a	163
	25. d	164
	26. c	155

Chapter 10

	Answer	Page reference
II.	1. *See text.*	
	2. Inhibits release of neurotransmitter substance P; inhibits conduction of pain impulses.	168
	3. *See text.*	171
	4. The intensity of the pain that a person is willing to endure before seeking relief	171
	5. Intensity of the stimulus necessary for the person to perceive pain	171
	6. Fatigue, anger, boredom, anxiety, persistent pain, illness.	171, *upper box; text*
	7. Meaning of pain to individual, degree of pain perception, past experience, cultural values, social expectations, physical and mental health, parental attitudes toward pain, setting in which pain occurs, fear and anxiety, usual way of responding to stressors, age.	171, *lower box; text*
	8. Pulse: increased rate Respirations: increased depth and frequency Blood pressure: increased systolic and diastolic Diaphoresis, pallor Dilated pupils Muscle tension (face, body) Nausea and vomiting (if pain is severe)	172
	9. *See Table 10-3.*	172
	10. P: Provoking factors: what makes the pain worse or relieves it Q: Quality: dull, sharp, crushing R: Region or radiation: site and radiation to other areas S: Severity or intensity T: Time: onset duration, frequency, cause	175

Chapter 10 (cont'd)

	Answer	Page reference
III.	1. b	170
	2. c	171
	3. b	171
	4. c	167
	5. b	168
	6. b	170
	7. d	173
	8. d	173
	9. b	175
	10. c	179-180
	11. a	180
	12. d	181
	13. d	183
	14. a	184
	15. d	168
	16. d	168
	17. b	178
	18. c	177
	19. d	178
	20. b	178
	21. b	171
	22. b	169
	23. a	174
	24. b	177
	25. c	183
	26. b	177
IV.	*See text.*	180
V.	*See text.*	178
VI.	*See text.*	177
VII.	1. *See text.*	170
	2. *See text.*	171
VIII.	1. Refer to McGuire, L: Seven myths about pain relief, RN 46:30-31, Dec 1983.	
	2. *See text.*	
	3. *Subjective answer.*	

Chapter 11

	Answer	Page reference
III.	1. b	190
	2. c	190
	3. a	190
	4. d	192
	5. b	193
	6. b	194
	7. d	191
	8. c	196
	9. c	194
	10. d	194

Chapter 11 (cont'd)

	Answer	Page reference
III.	11. c	194
	12. b	190
	13. a	197
	14. d	198
	15. c	201
	16. b	202
	17. d	202
	18. a	203
	19. d	204
	20. c	204
	21. b	209
	22. a	107
	23. a	209
	24. d	210
	25. c	210

Chapter 12

	Answer	Page reference
III.	1. d	215
	2. a	215
	3. c	
	4. d	227
	5. b	229
	6. b	245
	7. c	217-220
	8. c	220
	9. b	215
	10. d	218
	11. d	221
	12. b	219-220
	13. d	220-221
	14. a	225
	15. b	224
	16. c	225
	17. b	238-239
	18. c	250-251
VI.	1. a	255
	2. c	241
	3. a	241
	4. b	241
	5. a	240
	6. b	249
	7. d	249-250
	8. d	250
	9. a	253
	10. d	255-256
	11. a	257
	12. c	256
	13. a	224
	14. b	238-239
	15. c	253-254

Chapter 13

	Answer	Page reference
II.	1. c	265
	2. d	265
	3. f	265
	4. b	265
	5. e	265
	6. a	265
III.	1. b	274
	2. c	274
	3. a	274
IV.	1. a	277
	2. b	282
	3. d	282
	4. e	280
	5. c	279
	6. f	283
	7. b	282
	8. a	277
	9. e	280
	10. b	282
	11. c	279
	12. a	277
	13. f	283
	14. e	280
	15. b	282
	16. d	282
	17. f	283
	18. b	282
	19. f	283
V.	1. d	287
	2. c	264
	3. d	266
	4. a	266
	5. c	267
	6. a	267
	7. d	267
	8. a	268
	9. d	273
	10. d	275
	11. c	279
	12. a	277
	13. b	278
	14. c	279
	15. d	280
	16. d	283
	17. d	283
VI.	1. d	266
	2. f, g	266
	3. c	268
	4. h	268
	5. b	277
	6. a	281
	7. e	282

Chapter 14

	Answer	Page reference
III.	1. c	298
	2. c	302
	3. a	305
	4. a	292, 296
	5. c	297
	6. d	292
	7. c	292
	8. a	297
	9. a	298
	10. a	295
	11. d	299

Chapter 15

	Answer	Page reference
II.	Subjective responses	
III.	1. K	319-320
	2. M	319-320
	3. P	319-320
	4. M	319-320
	5. P	319-320
	6. K	319-320
	7. P	319-320
	8. K	319-320
	9. M	319-320
	10. M	319-320
IV.	1. c	315
	2. b	318
	3. a	322
	4. d	323
V.	1. F	315
	2. T	314
	3. T	314
	4. F	317
	5. F	318
	6. F	314
	7. T	321
	8. T	322
	9. F	324
	10. T	326
VI.	1. *See text.*	325
	2. *See text.*	325
	3. *See text.*	317
	4. *See text.*	326

Chapter 16

	Answer	Page reference
II.	1. d	332
	2. c	332
	3. d	333
	4. d	333
	5. a	335
	6. a	335
	7. b	337
	8. b	337, 340
	9. b	333
	10. d	342
III.	1. g	339
	2. c	341
	3. a	341
	4. f	341
	5. b	342
	6. d	344
	7. e	339

Answer

IV. Goals

1. Teach patient the correct procedure for turning, coughing, deep breathing, and leg exercises.
2. Teach patient the purpose and frequency of exercises.

Interventions

1. Instruct patient by demonstration and redemonstration using techniques in text, pp. 340-341, for deep breathing, coughing, leg exercises and turning.
2. Inform patient of purpose of postoperative exercises (see text pp. 340-341).

Evaluation

1. Patient returned demonstration correctly.
2. Patient verbalized purposes of postoperative exercises.

	Answer	Answer
V.	Across	Down
	1. Ectomy	5. Otomy
	2. Rrhaphy	6. Restorative
	3. Palliative	7. Curative
	4. Diagnostic	8. Scopy
	5. Ostomy	9. Plasty

Chapter 17

	Answer	Page reference
II.	1. Begins at the time the patient is transferred to the operating table and ends with transfer to the recovery area.	348
	2. *See table.*	349

Chapter 17 (cont'd)

	Answer	Page reference
II.	3. Primary surgeon Assistant to surgeon Scrub nurse	350
	4. Anesthesiologist Circulating nurse Other technicians Pathologist (if present)	350
	5. *See text.*	350
	6. *See text.*	350
	7. *See table and box.*	362, 363
	8. Excitability (laughing, crying, excessive talking), twitching, pulse or blood pressure changes, pallor of skin, respiratory difficulties.	364
	9. *See box.*	354

	Answer	Page reference
III.	1. f	356
	2. c	
	3. d	
	4. e	
	5. b	
	6. a	
IV.	1. c	349
	2. b	350
	3. b	356
	4. c	361
	5. b	364
	6. a	364
	7. c	364
	8. c	363
	9. b	360
	10. d	364
	11. a	355
	12. a	355
	13. c	354
V.	*See text.*	351

Chapter 18

Answer

II.

1. Airway obstruction; hypoventilation
2. a. Moving patient from O.R. table to bed
   b. Jarring in transport
   c. Loss of blood or body fluids, inadequate ventilation, cardiac arrythmias, cardiac failure, pain
3. a. Vital signs are stable
   b. Patient is awake and easily aroused
   c. Postsurgical complications are evaluated and under control
   d. Motor and partial sensory functions have returned to all anesthetized areas
4. a. Side rails up
   b. Call light in reach, instruct patient for permissability of ambulation or other activity
5. a. Respiratory status
   b. Circulatory status
   c. Neurological status
   d. Comfort
   e. Safety
   f. Equipment

Chapter 18 (cont'd)

	Answer	Page reference
III.	1. a	374
	2. b	374
	3. b	375
	4. d	375
	5. c	375
	6. d	373
	7. d	376
	8. b	376
	9. b	376
	10. b	376
	11. a	379
	12. a	379
	13. b	379
	14. a	387
	15. c	388
	16. d	388
	17. b	380
	18. b	381
	19. c	381
	20. a	383

Chapter 19

	Answer	Page reference
III.	1. c	407
	2. d	407
	3. a	407
	4. b	407
	5. a	407
IV.	Oxygen, carbon dioxide	403-404
	Proteins	403-404
	Potassium	403-404
	Sodium	403-404
	Polarized	403-404
	Sodium	403-404
	Positive	403-404
	Potassium	403-404
	Depolarization	403-404
	Repolarization	403-404
	Potassium	403-404
	Sodium	403-404
V.	1. a	400-401
	2. c	401-402
	3. d	402
	4. a and b	404
	5. c	414
	6. c	414
	7. d	415
	8. a	417
	9. b	452
	10. c	413 *(box)*
	11. c	421
	12. d	424

Chapter 19 (cont'd)

	Answer	Page reference
VI.	1. a	
	2. a	
	3. b	
	4. d	
	5. c	
VIII.	1. a	449-451
	2. c	451
	3. a	454
	4. d, c	454
	5. b	454
	6. c	463
	7. d	474
	8. c	475
	9. b	475
	10. a	476
	11. d	476
	12. d	476
	13. c	441
	14. b	485
	15. d	485
	16. a	480
X.	1. d	
	2. b	
	3. e	
	4. c	
	5. a	

XI. Brudzinski's sign
1, 5, 7
Babinski's sign
3, 8
Kernig's sign
1, 5, 6
Romberg's sign
2, 4, 9

	Answer	Answer
XII.	1. c	6. a
	2. c	7. a
	3. d	8. b
	4. c	9. d
	5. b	10. c

Answer

XIV.
1. fluent (sensory or receptive)
2. global
3. paraplegic
4. ptosis
5. papilledema
6. subarachnoid
7. dura
8. anisocoria
9. astereognosis
10. ataxia

Chapter 19 (cont'd)

	Answer	Page reference
XVI.	A. Decorticate	
	B. Decerebrate	
	C. Decorticate on right side of body; decerebrate on left side of body	
XVII.	1. Disorientation	
	2. Illusion	
	3. Hallucination	
	4. Vegetative state	
	5. Light coma	
XVIII.	1. b	419
	2. d	418, 419
	3. a	419
	4. d	448
	5. a	446
	6. d	469
	7. b	439
	8. c	441
	9. c	441
	10. b	441
	11. c	444
	12. b	444
	13. a	440
	14. c	439
	15. d	441
	16. a	441
	17. c	426
	18. b	419
	19. b	419
	20. a	419
	21. d	432
	22. a	426
	23. c	420
	24. b	432, 433
	25. a	437
XXI.	1. c	481-483
	2. a	481-483
	3. c	457
	4. a	457
	5. d	462
	6. a	455
	7. c	454
	8. d	477
	9. c	478-479
	10. a	487
	11. b	487
	12. b	487
	13. d	487
	14. b	441
	15. b	441
	16. d	437

Chapter 20

	Answer	Page reference
II.	*See text.*	517
III.	*See text.*	517
IV.	*See text.*	521

	Answer	Page reference
V.	1. a. Every 5 years	518
	b. Every 2 years	518
	2. By capillary attraction and by the upper lid	521
	3. 1 month to 3 months, because of the lack of blood vessels in cornea	532
	4. Prevent increased intraocular pressure; prevent stress on suture line; prevent hemorrhage in anterior chamber; prevent infection.	535
	5. Intracapsular	534
	6. Lens implant; contact lenses; cataract glasses.	535
	7. More acceptable to some elderly persons; no physical complications.	535
	8. 10-21 mm Hg	518
	9. Myopic degeneration; trauma; aphakia (absence of crystalline lens).	542
	10. Mydriatics will further restrict drainage of aqueous humor.	541
	11. Visual field no greater than 20 degrees central distance vision in better eye of 20/200.	525
	12. Anterior flexion of head; Straining or leaning over; lifting heavy objects; coughing.	535

	Answer	Page reference
VI.	1. i	519
	2. d	518
	3. g	520
	4. j	537
	5. c	520
	6. b	518
	7. e	516
	8. h	516
	9. f	519
	10. a	516

	Answer	Page reference
VII.	1. Regeneration of Rhodapsin in presence of vitamin A are in rods, which are receptors for dim or night visions.	516
	2. Intrinsic involuntary muscles	516
	3. 20/20	519
	4. Anyone with vision less than 20/30.	519
	5. Dilates pupil, blurs vision; do not drive, cannot read.	531
	6. Canal of Schlemm and ciliary muscle spaces.	518

	Answer	Page reference
VIII.	1. b	516
	2. a	516
	3. a	516
	4. d	516
	5. c	516
	6. a	518
	7. a	516
	8. b	519
	9. b	520
	10. d	516
	11. d	532
	12. b	532
	13. d	533

Chapter 20 (cont'd)

	Answer	Page reference
VIII.	14. b	533
	15. b	533
	16. a	535
	17. b	536
	18. a	539
	19. c	542
	20. d	543
	21. d	543
	22. c	526
	23. b	535
	24. a	535
	25. d	523
	26. b	519
	27. c	530
	28. b	531
	29. b	539
	30. a	529
	31. a	530
	32. d	524
	33. c	523
	34. a	528
	35. a	528
IX.	*See text.*	527

Answer **Page reference**

X. 537

Anterior chamber lens	Posterior chamber lens
In front of iris Extracapsular Attached flexible loops Extracapsular	Behind iris Intracapsular Ease of removal Small incision Rapid healing

	Answer	Page reference
XI.	1. a	537
	2. b	537
	3. b	537
	4. a	537
	5. a	537
	6. b	537
	7. b	537
	8. a	537
XII.	*See text.*	531

Chapter 21

	Answer	Page reference
II.	1. c	550
	2. a	
	3. b	
	4. d	

Chapter 21 (cont'd)

	Answer	Page reference
III.	1. Antibiotics	551
	Diuretics	
	Salicylates	
	2. Pain	553
	Hearing loss	
	3. Boric acid and alcohol	555
	4. Hydrogen peroxide	555
	5. *See chart.*	556
	6. 1. Antivert	558
	2. Dramamine	
	3. Benadryl	
	4. Hydrodiuril	
	5. Nicotinic acid	
IV.	1. d	557
	2. a	557
	3. b	564
	4. b	556
	5. d	555
	6. c	555
	7. b	565
	8. c	565
	9. d	563
	10. a	558
	11. d	562
	12. b	549
	13. d	550
	14. a	550
	15. a	550
	16. b	554
V.	1. *See chart.*	556
	2. *See box.*	560
VI.	*See box.*	563

Chapter 22

	Answer	Page reference
II.	1. *See text.*	572-573
	2.	574
	3.	576
	4.	574
III.	1. *See text.*	577-581
	2.	580-587
	3.	591-596
	4.	600
	5.	601-604
	6.	619-624
IV.	1. c	612
	2. f	612
	3. e	612
	4. a	612
	5. d	612
	6. b	612

Chapter 22 (cont'd)

	Answer	Page reference
V.	1. c	577
	2. a	576
	3. d	577
	4. c	577
	5. a	577
	6. d	578
	7. a	578
	8. c	579
	9. c	581
	10. d	581
	11. b	582
	12. d	594
	13. b	595
	14. a	607
	15. d	607
	16. c	588
	17. a	627
	18. b	624
	19. d	621
	20. c	622
	21. a	629
	22. d	629-630
	23. a	613
	24. c	615-616
	25. d	618
	26. d	618
	27. d	619
	28. a	624
	29. c	623
	30. d	616

Chapter 23

	Answer	Page reference
II.	*See table.*	640
III.	1. b	642
	2. c	
	3. a	
	4. d	
IV.	1. b	640
	2. b	645
	3. b	646
	4. d	647
	5. b	649
	6. a	651
	7. c	645-651
	8. a	653
	9. d	653
	10. c	659
	11. c	649
	12. c	649-650

Chapter 23 (cont'd)

	Answer	Page reference
VI.	1. *See box.*	645
	2. *See box.*	651

	Answer	Page reference
VI.	1. It may be associated with nasal polyposis.	643
	2. Avoid: chilling, air conditioning when outside air is warm and moist, smoking, fatigue, others with infections; protect nose during swimming; avoid diving.	643
	3. Trauma, chronic infection, lack of humidity in air breathed, violent sneezing or noseblowing, nose picking (most common cause).	648
VII.	1. Wash hands. 2. Tip head backward. 3. Turn head to side that will receive the drops. 4. Place no more than 3 drops of solution into each nostril. 5. Remain in position with head tilted backward for 5 minutes. 6. If marked congestion is still present, another drop or two of solution may be administered.	641

Chapter 24

	Answer	Page reference
II.	1. Provide oxygen to cells; remove excess carbon dioxide from cells.	666
	2. Adequate supply of oxygen in the environment; a patent airway; normally functioning bellow motion of the chest wall and diaphragm; an adequate number of functioning alveoli and capillaries that together form a terminal respiratory unit (TRU); adequate amount of hemoglobin to carry oxygen to the cells; intact circulatory system and an effective heart pump; and a functioning respiratory center.	668
	3. Eat a balanced diet; get adequate rest and sleep; avoid crowds during times of prevalent infections; get appropriate immunizations.	670
	4. Chronic cough, sputum, dyspnea.	671
	5. Chronic bronchitis, emphysema, asthma	671
	6. Vesicular, localized rales, sibilant rhonchi.	674
	7. *See box.*	681
	8. New York, California, Texas, Florida.	683
	9. Encourage fluids, collect specimens before meals, rinse mouth before collection, send to lab immediately.	686
	10. *See box.*	734

	Answer	Page reference
III.	A. 1. b 2. a 3. d 4. c	675
	B. 1. c 2. a 3. d 4. e 5. f 6. b	705
IV.	1. c	666-667
	2. b	666-704
	3. c	667
	4. b	669
	5. d	674
	6. c	679
	7. c	686
	8. d	686
	9. d	686

Chapter 24 (cont'd)

	Answer	Page reference
IV.	10. c	697
	11. a	699-701
	12. b	667
	13. b	704
	14. c	707
	15. c	709
	16. a	714
	17. b	722
	18. d	722
	19. d	723
	20. b	725
	21. c	725
	22. c	733
	23. d	733
	24. b	735
	25. c	743
	26. a	743
	27. b	744
	28. c	744
V.	1. *See chart.*	697
	2. *See box.*	709
	3. *See Care Plan.*	738, 739
	4. *See Care Plan.*	748-750

Chapter 25

	Answer	Page reference
II.	1. *See illustrations.*	759
	2. *See illustrations.*	756
III.	1. *See text.*	756
	2.	756
	3.	759
	4.	759
	5.	760
	6.	759
IV.	1. b	759
	2. c	759
	3. b	760
	4. c	756
	5. c	760
	6. c	760
V.	SA node AV node Bundle of His Right and left bundle branches Purkinje's fibers	
VII.		759

Chapter 25 (cont'd)

	Answer	Answer	Page reference
VIII.	*Across*	*Down*	765
	1. Pulse pressure	1. p	
	2. Myocardium	3. Conductivity	
	3. Cardiac Output	9. Endocardium	764, Fig. 25-9
	4. Epicardium	10. Preload	
	5. Automaticity	11. Septum	
	6. Diastolic	12. Afterload	
	7. Orthopnea	13. Systolic	
	8. Excitability	14. HDL	

	Answer	Page reference
IX.	1. f	
	2. c	
	3. a	
	4. e	
	5. d	
	6. b	
X.	1. 120	764-765
	2. 0.12	764-765
	3. 6.64	764-765
	4. Regular	764-765
	5. Yes	764-765
	6. Yes	764-765
	7. b	764-765
XI.	1. c	766
	2. d	769
	3. a	767
	4. a	766
	5. c	766
	6. d	768
	7. a	767
	8. a	766
	9. b	761
	10. c	760
	11. a	760
	12. d	773
	13. b	774
XII.	T, P	
	T, P	
	P	
XIX.	1. b	779, *box.*
	2. b	778
	3. c	781, *Table 25-4*
	4. c	784, *box.*
	5. d	788
	6. a	792
	7. a	786
	8. c	788, *box;* 797, *box.*
	9. a	802
	10. b	*See Chapter 13, pp. 269-272, 274-275.*
	11. d	795
	12. b	798, *Fig. 25-3.*
	13. c	799, *box.*
	14. b	799

Chapter 25 (cont'd)

	Answer	Page reference
XIX.	15. b	799
	16. a	799-800
	17. c	797, *box.*
	18. a	800
	19. c	802

Chapter 26

	Answer	Page reference
II.	1. Cigarette smoking	828-830
	Hypertension	828-830
	Hyperlipidemia	828-830
	Obesity	828-830
	Physical inactivity	828-830
	Emotional stress	828-830
	Diabetes mellitus	828-830
	2. Heparin and coumadin	836
	3. *See box.*	851
	4. *See text.*	854
	5. *See table.*	837
	6. Vitamin K	837
III.	1. b	835-836
	2. a	835-836
	3. c	835-836
	4. e	835-836
	5. d	835-836
IV.	*See table.*	855
V.	1. d	347
	2. a	850
	3. b	836
	4. a	842
	5. d	847
	6. b	830
	7. b	831
	8. a	832
	9. b	832
	10. c	834
	11. b	847
	12. c	830
	13. b	855
	14. a	856
	15. a	828
	16. d	847
	17. b	855
VI.	*See text.*	855

Chapter 27

	Answer	Page reference
II.	1. The blood and its components, reticuloendothelial system.	864
	2. Red blood cells (erythrocytes), white blood cells (leukocytes), platelets (thrombocytes).	
	3. Phagocytosis	866

Chapter 27 (cont'd)

	Answer	Page reference
II.	4. Blood loss, impaired RBC production, hemolysis, nutritional deficiency.	868 *(chart)*
	5. Liver, egg yolk, dried fruit, dark green, leafy vegetables, whole grains.	881 *(box)*

	Answer	Page reference
III.	1. b	883
	2. a	883
	3. d	883
	4. c	883
IV.	*See table.*	870-871
V.	1. c	865
	2. d	865
	3. a	865
	4. b	865
	5. d	868
	6. b	868
	7. c	871
	8. c	883
	9. a	883
	10. c	885
	11. d	887
	12. b	889-893
	13. a	889
	14. b	891
	15. d	892
	16. c	894
	17. a	894
	18. a	872
	19. c	873
	20. b	873
	21. c	874
	22. a	874
	23. a	881
	24. a	883
VI.	*See Care Plan.*	876-879

Chapter 28

	Answer	Page reference
II.	1. Lowers blood glucose	904
	2. *See table.*	905
	3. *See chart.*	906
	4. Primary: Maintain ideal weight, genetic counseling. Secondary: Screening programs, health education.	907-909
	5. *See table.*	908
	6. Weakness Nervousness Perspiration Mental confusion	925
	7. Polydipsia Polyuria Polyphagia Weight loss Fatigue	909

Chapter 28 (cont'd)

	Answer	Page reference
II.	8. *See chart.*	910-911
	9. Protein: 12%-20%; carbohydrate: 55%-60%; fat: 30%.	916
	10. Legumes, oats, barley, fruit.	916
	11. Milk products, vegetables, fruit, starch/bread, meat, fats.	917

	Answer	Page reference
III.	1. a	920
	2. c	
	3. b	
	4. d	
IV.	1. b	934-935
	2. c	905
	3. d	905
	4. d	911
	5. a	909
	6. a	911
	7. d	910
	8. c	910
	9. b	917-919
	10. c	907
	11. b	913
	12. a	913
	13. c	913
	14. d	913
	15. c	915
	16. d	936-938
	17. a	906-907
	18. b	913
	19. b	936-938
	20. b	919
	21. d	920
	22. a	920
	23. b	920
	24. c	918
	25. b	910-911
	26. a	907
	27. b	912
	28. a	914
	29. c	919
	30. b	925
	31. c	924
V.	1. *See chart.*	919
	2. *See chart.*	919
	3. *See chart.*	925-926

Chapter 29

	Answer	Page reference
II.	1. Pituitary, adrenal, thyroid, parathyroid.	942
	2. *See table.*	943
	3. Glucocorticoids (cortisol), mineralocorticoids (aldosterone).	944
	4. Epinephrine, norepinephrine.	944
	5. Coughing, sneezing, blowing the nose, bending over, straining.	956
	6. Hypotension, dehydration, hyponatremia, hyperkalemia, hypoglycemia.	956
	7. Paresthesia, Chvostek's sign, Trousseau's sign, carpopedal spasm.	972

Chapter 29 (cont'd)

	Answer	Page reference
III.	1. c	943
	2. b	942
	3. d	942
	4. a	946
	5. c	967
	6. d	943
	7. c	956
	8. a	958
	9. b	965
	10. a	968
	11. a	968
	12. a	975
	13. a	978
IV.	*See box.*	957

Chapter 30

	Answer	Page reference
II.	1. Carbohydrate, protein, and fat metabolism; production of bile salts; bilirubin metabolism; detoxification of substances; storage of minerals and vitamins.	993
	2. Abdominal tenderness, rebound tenderness, muscle rigidity or spasm, decreased or absent bowel signs, abdominal distention.	1001
	3. *See illustrations.*	1013-1014
	4. *See text.*	1016
	5. Intolerance of fatty foods, flatus, nausea and vomiting, pain in right upper quadrant, diarrhea, abdominal distention.	1030
	6. Pain, nausea and vomiting, abdominal distention, steatorrhea, polyuria, polydipsia, polyphagia, weight loss, fever.	1041

	Answer	Page reference
III.	*See chart.*	998
IV.	1. b	993
	2. c	994
	3. b	996
	4. a	996
	5. d	997
	6. d	999-1000
	7. c	1001
	8. b	1001
	9. d	1001
	10. d	1002
	11. a	1008
	12. c	1011
	13. d	1011
	14. c	1012
	15. b	1015
	16. d	1016
	17. d	1016
	18. b	1018-1019
	19. d	1032
	20. a	1038
	21. a	1038
V.	1. *See Care Plan.*	1007-1009
	2. *See box.*	1026-1027

Chapter 31

	Answer	Page reference
II.	1. a	1048
	2. b	1048
	3. b	1048
	4. b	1048
	5. b	1056
	6. a	1056
	7. a	1057
	8. b	1063
	9. b	1075
	10. b	1075 *(Table)*
	11. c	1075
	12. d	1077
	13. d	1079
	14. c	1074
	15. d	1080
	16. a	1071
	17. c	1077, 1067
	18. a	1082
	19. b	1082
	20. a	1074
	21. c	1096
	22. a	1085
	23. d	1085
	24. c	1085
	25. b	1085
	26. a	1083
	27. a	1095
	28. b	1069
	29. b	1070
	30. b	1070
	31. a	1085
	32. c	1085
	33. b	1085
	34. a	1085
	35. a	1102
	36. b	1080
	37. c	1102
III.	1. d	
	2. b	1061
	3. a	1059
	4. b	1054
	5. f	1083
	6. c	
	7. e	1054
	8. g	
IV.	1. d	1105, *Table 31-21.*
	2. c	1094
	3. a	1094
	4. b	1105
	5. Jejunum Duodenum Ileum	1048
	6. Cecum Colon Rectum	1048

Chapter 31 (cont'd)

	Answer	Page reference
VI.	1. A mass. The mass can be in the groin, umbilicus, scrotum, or from an old incision. The mass may be present all the time or appear suddenly after coughing, straining, sneezing, lifting, or other vigorous exercises.	1104
	2. Surgery	1104
	3. —Report signs of wound infection —Ice bags to scrotum if edema still present —Explain that sexual functioning is not altered —No driving for 2 weeks —Avoid heavy lifting, pulling, physical exertion, and constipation	1104
	4. There is a high incidence of cancer associated with polyposis. The majority of these lesions are malignant.	1105, *table.*
	5. —Low-residue diet about 3-4 days before surgery; then clear liquids for 2-3 days before surgery Neomycin or erythromycin —Enemas —Laxatives	
	6. High-fiber	1094
	7. Bolic forms of oral medications are not absorbed. Only liquid or chewable forms of oral medications should be given.	1100, *box*
	8. Avoid high-fiber or high-residue foods after surgery. Then gradually add one of the high-fiber types of foods to tolerance. If unable to tolerate, eliminate from diet.	
	9. Usually none. Most patients, however, will avoid gas-forming foods.	1115
	10. The purpose of colostomy irrigations is to regulate the bowels.	1114
	11. Take no action. This is normal. Flatus and fecal drainage normally begin within 2-3 days following an ileostomy and 4-7 days following a colostomy.	1114
	12. Initially both stomas will have a mucous and serosanguineous type drainage.	1111
	13. Skin irritation, blockage from food, prolapse of stoma, and stricture of stoma. An additional problem specific for the colostomy is constipation.	1116, *box*
	14. Red, moist, slightly edematous	
	15. Yes	

	Answer
VII.	1. d
	2. g
	3. f
	4. h
	5. c
	6. a
	7. b
	8. e
	9. i

	Answer	Page reference
VIII.	1. b	1087-1088
	2. d	1088
	3. b	1088
	4. c	1088
	5. a	1087
	6. a	1089
	7. d	1091
	8. d	1091
	9. a	1091
	10. c	1091
	11. c	1094
	12. a	1094
	13. c	1097
	14. a	1098

Chapter 31 (cont'd)

	Answer	Page reference
VIII.	15. d	1097, 1099
	16. d	1117
	17. d	1119
	18. b	1119
	19. d	1102
	20. c	1103
	21. c	1104
	22. a	1108
	23. b	1108
	24. a	1111

CASE STUDY

Answer	Page reference
1. Tell patient that a tube will be passed through the mouth to the stomach to view the inside of the stomach and remove a small piece of tissue for examination. He will not be allowed to have anything to eat or drink after midnight. Have patient sign a consent for the procedure. Explain that medication will be given intravenously to sedate him immediately before the procedure. The procedure will take place in a special lab and will take about 1 hour. Let him know that he may have a sore throat after the procedure. Explain that an anesthetic agent will be sprayed in his throat to relax the throat for easier passage of the tube.	1074, *box.*
2. Do not give anything to eat or drink until gag reflex returns. Monitor vital signs. If patient complains of sore throat, give warm saline gargles or obtain order for an analgesic throat spray.	1074, *box.*
3. The nurse should measure and record the amount of solution used to irrigate the N/G tube, then subtract the total amount of solution used for irrigation from the total amount of N/G drainage.	1069, *lower box.*
4. Seek clarification by saying, "A matter of time before what happens?" The statement by Mr. Provost is one that is commonly made by patients who are faced with dying. Allow Mr. Provost to ventilate his feelings about death and dying.	*See Chapter 15.*

Chapter 32

	Answer	Page reference
II.	1. *See illustration.*	1125
	2. a. 5	1126-1228
	b. 12	1126-1228
	c. 2	1126-1228
	d. 8	1126-1228
	e. 1	1126-1228
	f. 3	1126-1228
	g. 10	1126-1228
	h. 6	1126-1228
	i. 4	1126-1228
	j. 9	1126-1228
	k. 7	1126-1228
	l. 11	1126-1228
	3. *See illustration.*	1128
	4. *See illustration.*	1124
	5. *See illustration.*	1125

Chapter 32 (cont'd)

	Answer	Page reference
III.	Detrusor	1128
	Relaxing	1128
	150-350	1128
	Parasympathetic	1128
	Stimulated	1128
	Afferent	1128
	Afferent	1128
	Contraction	1128
	Internal	1128
	Relaxation	1128
	External	1128
IV.	*See text.*	
V.	*See text.*	
VI.	1. d	1132
	2. b	1133
	3. c	1135
	4. c	1136
	5. c	1141
	6. b	1137
	7. c	1166
	8. c	1139
	9. c	1144
	10. b	1150
	11. a	1148
	12. a	1151
	13. c	1153
	14. d	1153
	15. a	1154
	16. b	1155
	17. c	1157
	18. a	1144
	19. d	1186
	20. b	1145
	21. c	1183
	22. b	1158
	23. c	1161
	24. c	1161
	25. b	1169
	26. a	1169
	27. d	1174
	28. d	1174
	29. d	1185
	30. b	1186
	31. a	1189
	32. c	1190
	33. c	1188
	34. b	1132
	35. c	1192
	36. b	1192
	37. d	1210
	38. d	1210
	39. a	1211
	40. a	1212

Chapter 32 (cont'd)

	Answer	Page reference
VI.	41. b	1212
	42. d	1212
	43. d	1212
	44. b	1124
	45. a	1124
	46. a	1133
	47. c	1127
	48. d	1127
	49. a	1131
	50. b	1134
	51. a	1132
	52. c	1149
	53. b	1135

Chapter 33

	Answer	Page reference
II.	1. b	1220
	2. c	1221
	3. a	1221
	4. a	1221
	5. a	1221
	6. b	1221
	7. b	1221
	8. b	1223
	9. c	1223
	10. a	1225
	11. d	1226
	12. c	1228
	13. d	1228
	14. a	1228
	15. a	1228
	16. b	1233
	17. d	1229
	18. b	1229
	19. d	1229-1230
	20. a	1230
	21. d	1230
	22. c	1230
	23. d	1231
	24. a	1231
	25. b	1232

Chapter 34

	Answer	Page reference
III.	1. c	1240
	2. d	1240
	3. a	1241
	4. c	1244
	5. c	1245
	6. a	1241
	7. b	1266
	8. d	1246
	9. d	1247
	10. b	1248

Chapter 34 (cont'd)

	Answer	Page reference
III.	11. c	1249
	12. c	1249
	13. a	1250
	14. d	1252
	15. a	1253
	16. d	1253
	17. b	1254
	18. a	1253
	19. c	1253
	20. b	1256
	21. a	1260
	22. c	1261
	23. b	1261
	24. d	1263
	25. d	1264
	26. a	1264
	27. d	1265
	28. b	1266
	29. c	1271

Chapter 35

	Answer	Page reference
I.	1. c	1280
	2. d	1280-1281
	3. a	1281
	4. a	1281
	5. b	1284
	6. d	1283
	7. c	1288
	8. a	1282
	9. a	1293
	10. b	1293

Chapter 36

Answer

I. *Oophorectomy*—removal of ovaries
Gynecomasia—overdevelopment of breast tissue (males)
Orange peel effect—the thickening and dimpling effect of the skin that overlays malignant tumors of the breast
Mastitis—Infection of breast tissue
ERA—Estrogen receptor assay test to determine presence of estrogen dependent tumors
Fibroadenomas—fibroplastic tumors commonly seen in young women under 25

	Answer	Page reference
II.	1. b	1304
	2. c	1305
	3. d	1304
	4. a	1304
	5. c	1304
	6. b	1309
	7. c	1312
	8. d	1313
	9. a	1317
	10. b	1317

Chapter 36 (cont'd)

	Answer	Page reference
II.	11. a	1307
	12. b	1312-1313
	13. a	1313
	14. d	1313
	15. a	1311
	16. c	1319
	17. a	1310
	18. d	1310
	19. d	1306
	20. d	1310
	21. a	1310
	22. a	1304
	23. b	1304
	24. a	1304
	25. c	1311

Chapter 37

	Answer	Page reference
II.	1. Skin; blood protein or blood pH; proteins: interferon, immogloblins; lymph nodes, thymus gland; WBC and phagacytes.	1331-1338
	2. Active immunity	1331
	3. Plasma	1334
	4. Interferon is produced by certain virally infected cells. It functions as a defense mechanism by protecting uninfected cells from viral multiplication.	1335
	5. Vascular, fluid exudation, cellular exudation	1337
	6. Thymus	1342
	7. Redness, heat, swelling, pain, loss of function	1337
	8. *See text.*	1330
	9. From prior contact with the antigen or through introduction of specifically protective antibodies or cells inside the body	1330

	Answer	Page reference
III.	1. a	1331
	2. c	1331
	3. b	1331
	4. d	1331
IV.	1. b	1331
	2. a	1331
	3. d	1331
	4. c	1331
V.	1. T	1340-1341
	2. B	1340-1341
	3. T	1340-1341
	4. T	1340-1341
	5. B	1340-1341
	6. B	1340-1341
	7. T	1340-1341
	8. B	1340-1341
	9. T	1340-1341
	10. T	1340-1341

Chapter 37 (cont'd)

	Answer	Page reference
VI.	1. b	1337
	2. b	1339
	3. c	1338
	4. a	1344
	5. d	1343
	6. b	1335
	7. d	1334
	8. b	1330
	9. c	1338
	10. d	1339
	11. b	1333
	12. d	1335
VII.	1. *See details of mechanisms.*	1330
	2. *See inflammatory response.*	1337

Chapter 38

	Answer	Page reference
II.	1. Concentrated solution of antibodies	1357
	2. ELISA and Western blot test	1360
	3. Responsiveness of host, increased amount of allergen, nature of allergen, entrance of allergen into body, short time period between contacts.	1363
III.	1. A-A, O B-B, O AB-A, B, AB, O O-O	1367
	2. Type O	1367
	3. Type AB	1367
IV.	A. *See text.*	1370
	B. *See text.*	1371
	C. *See table.*	1365
V.	1. Protein-calorie malnutrition, alcoholism, infections, cancer, autoimmune diseases, lymphomas, allergies, trauma, transplantation.	1355
	2. Constricts smooth muscle	1363-1364
	Increases vascular permeability	1364
	Increases mucous secretions	1364
	3. The presence of antigen Rh-D is implied	1369
	Indicates the absence of antigen D	1369

	Answer	Page reference
VI.	1. a	1362-1372
	2. d	1362-1372
	3. a	1362-1372
	4. c	1362-1372
	5. b	1362-1372
	6. d	1362-1372
	7. a	1362-1372
	8. d	1362-1372

Chapter 38 (cont'd)

	Answer	Page reference
VII.	1. b	1356
	2. d	1357
	3. a	1360
	4. b	1360
	5. c	1362
	6. b	1364
	7. d	1366
	8. c	1366
	9. c	1366

	Answer	Page reference
VIII.	1. A retrovirus (HIV)	1357
	2. Sexual contact, infection of contaminated needles, mother to fetus.	1357
	3. 6-12 weeks	1360
	4. Homosexual and bisexual men with multiple contacts, IV drug users.	1357
	5. ELISA	1360
	6. *See text.*	1358
	7. Pneumonia Kaposi's sarcoma	1359
	8. *See text.*	1358

Chapter 39

	Answer	Page reference
II.	1. Protection, heat regulation, sensory perception, excretion, production of vitamin D.	1379
	2. Griseofulvin	1382
	3. Pediculosis: head lice Pediculosis: body lice Pediculosis: pubic lice Scabies	1383
	4. Kaposi's sarcoma	1398
	5. Full-thickness graft	1400
	6. *See text.*	1400

	Answer	Page reference
III.	*See Data analysis.*	1381-1382
IV.	*See table.*	1383
V.	*See text.*	1385
VI.	1. a	1378
	2. d	1384
	3. d	1384
	4. a	1399
	5. a	1400
	6. b	1403
	7. a	1403
	8. b	1395, 1397
	9. d	1381
	10. d	1383
	11. c	1380
	12. d	1389
	13. d	1389

Chapter 39 (cont'd)

	Answer	Page reference
VII.	1. c	1395
	2. d	1395
	3. a	1395
	4. b	1395
	5. e	1395
VIII.	1. *See Care Plan.*	1387
	2. *See Care Plan.*	1401

Chapter 40

	Answer	Page reference
II.	1. Emergent, acute, rehabilitative.	1412
	2. "Rule of Nines"	1413
	3. Elderly (or, those over 60 years of age) Very young (or, those under two years of age)	1413-1414
	4. Size and depth of the burn, age of the victim, body part involved, burning agent, medical history.	1413-1416
	5. May choose from several answers; *see text.*	1423-1426
	6. Exercising, splinting, and applying pressure dressings.	1435
	7. Protein	1429
	8. Homografts Heterografts	1426
	9. Contractures	1431-1432
	10. *See table.*	1424-1426

	Answer	Page reference
III.	1. d	1417-1418
	2. a	1410
	3. c	1411
	4. c	1419
	5. c	1418
	6. b	1409
	7. c	1410-1411
	8. a	1418
	9. c	1410
	10. c	1409
	11. d	1409-1410
	12. d	1426
	13. a	1426
	14. c	1430
	15. b	1428
	16. a	1429
	17. c	1432

CASE STUDY

	Answer	Page reference
	See text.	1409, 1413, 1414, 1418, 1419

Chapter 41

	Answer	Page reference
II.	*See chart.*	1455
III.	*See chart.*	1456

Chapter 41 (cont'd)

	Answer	Page reference
IV.	1. b	1446
	2. a	1447
	3. b	1454
	4. c	1459
	5. d	1459
	6. c	1460
	7. d	1460
	8. b	1461
	9. c	1454
	10. b	1448
	11. d	1453
	12. a	1447
	13. b	1446
	14. d	1447
V.	1. *See details of assessment.*	1453
	2. *See details of assessment.*	1453
	3. *See details of assessment.*	1448, 1449
	4. *See details of assessment.*	1450

Chapter 42

	Answer	Page reference
II.	1. *See text.*	1480-1481
	2. Mechanical ventilation	1482
	3. Bleeding, thrombosis, inflammation/infiltration, infection, air embolism, paresthesias, distal obstruction of artery.	1475
	4. Arrhythmias, infection, intracardiac knotting, thrombophlebitis, balloon rupture with air embolism, pulmonary artery rupture, pulmonary infarction.	1477
	5. Dyspnea, chest pain, fever, hemoptysis, tachycardia, pleural friction rub.	1486
	6. Aids in expanding alveoli, preventing further collapse; improving oxygen transport.	1482
	7. Maintain patent airway, minimize arterial blood gas changes, oxygenate patient before and after suctioning, limit suctioning to 15 seconds, elevate head of bed 30 degrees (facilitates venous drainage without impeding arterial supply), maintain head and neck in straight alignment, prevent overly tight tracheostomy ties, prevent valsalva maneuver, assist patient in turning, prevent coughing, sneezing, constipation, monitor hydration status intake and output.	1484
	8. *See box.*	1485
	9. Cimetidine (Tagamet)	1486

	Answer	Page reference
III.	1. g	1477 *table.*
	2. d	
	3. a	
	4. c	
	5. f	
	6. e	
	7. b	
IV.	*See table.*	1483
V.	1. b	1476
	2. a	1476
	3. b	1475
	4. a	1475
	5. d	1482

Chapter 42 (cont'd)

	Answer	Page reference
V.	6. a	1482
	7. a	1480
	8. b	1472
	9. c	1477
	10. a	1482
	11. a	1482
	12. b	1477
	13. a	1485
	14. c	1485
	15. c	1478-1479
VI.	*See box.*	1474
	See complete assessment and interventions.	1486-1490